CANCER
PREVENTION
MADE EASY

ROBERT G. SCHNEIDER, M.D.

CANCER PREVENTION MADE EASY

Prentice-Hall, Inc., Englewood Cliffs, New Jersey 07632

Library of Congress Cataloging in Publication Data

Schneider, Robert G. (date)
    Cancer prevention made easy.

    Bibliography: p.
    Includes index.
    1. Cancer—Diet therapy.   2. Cancer—Prevention.
3. Carotenes—Therapeutic use.   I. Title.
RC271.D52S36 1984   616.99'4052   83-27024
ISBN 0-13-113994-0

ISBN 0-13-113994-0

Editorial/production supervision by Elizabeth Torjussen
Jacket design © 1984 by Jeannette Jacobs
Manufacturing buyer: Pat Mahoney

This book is available at a special discount when ordered in
bulk quantities. Contact Prentice-Hall, Inc., General
Publishing Division, Special Sales, Englewood Cliffs, N.J. 07632.

Prentice-Hall International, Inc., *London*
Prentice-Hall of Australia Pty. Limited, *Sydney*
Prentice-Hall Canada Inc., *Toronto*
Prentice-Hall of India Private Limited, *New Delhi*
Prentice-Hall of Japan, Inc., *Tokyo*
Prentice-Hall of Southeast Asia Pte. Ltd., *Singapore*
Whitehall Books Limited, *Wellington, New Zealand*
Editora Prentice-Hall do Brasil Ltda., *Rio de Janeiro*

For our children,
who refuse to eat vegetables
. . . but we're working on it.

I look for the end of cancer before this century is over. I now believe it could begin to fall in place at almost any time, starting next year or even next week. . . .

Dr. Lewis Thomas, Chancellor
Memorial Sloan–Kettering Cancer Center
New York City

CONTENTS

THE CANCER RISK TEST

Score-Yourself Checklist

A. Factors that *increase* your risk		Points	Your Score
Tobacco	1–10	1	
cigarettes per day	11–20	2	
	21–40	3	
	over 40	5	_____
Alcohol	2–3	1	
drinks per day	4–5	2	
	over 5	3	_____
Tobacco *and* Alcohol		1	
any amount			_____
Animal Fat (Red Meat)	2–3	1	
steak, hamburger, etc.	4–5	3	
times per week	over 5	5	_____
Animal Fat (Dairy)	2–3	1	
whole milk, butter, cheese, cream, etc.	4–5	3	
times per week	over 5	5	_____
Smoked Foods	over 1	1	
times per week			
Pickled Foods	over 1	1	
times per week			_____
Foods Preserved with Nitrites	over 1	1	
(bacon, sausage, bologna, etc.)			
times per week			_____
Charcoal Broiling	over 1	1	
times per week			_____
Frying at Prolonged High Heat	over 1	1	
times per week			_____
Overweight (over 10%)		1	
see Weight Table in Chapter 12			_____
Sun Worshipper		1	_____
X-Ray Exams or Therapy		1	
many, especially in childhood			_____
Occupational Exposure		1	
asbestos, chemicals, pollutants, etc.			_____
Drugs		1	
e.g., estrogen (post-menopausal)			_____
Viruses		1	
e.g., genital herpes			_____
Chronic Irritation Diseases		1	
e.g., ulcerative colitis			_____
		Total Points	_____

B. Factors that *decrease* your risk

		Points	
Beta Carotene Vegetables	1–3	2	
see list Chapter 16	4–6	4	
portions per week	7 plus	6	_____
Citrus Fruits	3–6	1	
portions per week	7 plus	2	_____
Grains and Cereals	3–6	1	
portions per week	7 plus	2	_____
Fiber (Vegetables and Whole Grains)	3–6	1	
portions per week	7 plus	2	_____
		Total Points	_____

A minus B equals your Cancer Risk Score _____

Compare your score: Less than 3 = Low Risk

3 to 6 = Moderate Risk

More than 6 = High Risk

You *can* lower your risk and increase your lifespan! Read on.

CANCER AND DIET

ONE

CANCER IS PREVENTABLE

Cancer is *not* an inevitable, unavoidable consequence of aging. Cancer, like heart disease, is preventable. The realization that we are not at the mercy of our own bodies, that life and health are not a giant lottery, comes as a happy shock and a gratifying surprise, after my years as a practicing physician. Put to use the new knowledge about cancer—it is so simple, it's jawdropping. Otherwise, resign yourself to accepting cancer as the irrational whimsy of fate. There is a signpost at a fork in the road: You, the reader, choose every day of your life which route you will take, whether or not you are aware of it. Now a roadmap is provided.

As a doctor devoted to preventive medicine, I preach tumor prevention to the patients I see in my practice of internal medicine and cardiology, but until now only odd fragments were known: the relationship between smoking and cancer, asbestos exposure and mesothelioma of the lung, sunlight and skin melanoma, radiation and leukemia, chemicals (for example, PCBs: polychlorinated biphenyls) and tumors. What has opened my eyes wide with hope and expectation is the emergence of what I am now calling the Unified Concept of Cancer Prevention, a new era signifying relief from the nightmare of cancer.

What you will learn from reading this book may be new, but is deeply rooted in the history of primitive mankind. Food for thought: prevention of heart disease, hypertension (high blood pressure), diabetes, and obesity jibes provocatively with cancer prevention. These lethal diseases are all caused in part by parallel errors in modern nutrition.

Between them, cardiovascular disease and cancer account for 70 to 80 percent of all deaths in the United States. With the number-one and -two killers under control, we can begin to imagine the limits intrinsic in our genes. Perhaps one hundred years, or even the biblical one hundred and twenty years, of physically and mentally vigorous life are written on our blueprint, not to mention the uncharted potential of genetic engineering.

Does it sound a little too much like the colorful nineteenth-century medicine man rolling into a dusty prairie village, his horse and wagon decorated with promises of miracle cures, to sell quack remedies to gullible citizens? But we are not talking about dousing ourselves with Kickapoo tonic juice or wahoo Indian remedies for scrofula, quinsy, or lumbago. That romantic fantasy, as you will read, is coalescing at this moment into reality under the critical gaze of demanding scientists. Within a decade or two the need for radical surgery, tissue-incinerating radiation therapy, and bone-marrow-destroying chemotherapy (drugs) to treat cancer may seem as primitive as bloodletting for fevers, cupping to draw out evil humors and vapors, or wearing garlic-filled amulets around the neck to ward off contagion.

This is what I propose to show in this book:

1. What is cancer?
2. What causes cancer? We now know the cause of 90 percent of all cancers.
3. How to prevent cancer. Eighty percent of cancers are preventable.
4. The crucial role of diet, the single most important factor. Forty percent of male cancers and 60 percent of female cancers are diet related. What foods *cause* cancer and what foods *prevent* cancer. Overweight as a major cancer risk factor.
5. In addition to food, what the other preventable causes of cancer are and how to cope with them.
6. What's wrong with the nationally publicized popular diets. Why low-carbohydrate or high-protein diets, counting grams or calories, and all the other twists and turns in the nutritional maze can lead you astray.
7. A practical guide to managing your own cancer prevention program: food groups, food lists, quantities, preparation, menus, and recipes.

No complex lists, sheets, or books to carry around with you. No need to consult rumpled papers furtively concealed in your lap under the edge of the tablecloth when dining out.

8. The seven key words: Have you had your beta unit today?
9. What is a beta unit?
10. Answers to questions.

You can read the book through from page 1 or you can skip around, focusing on those parts that interest you most.

If you want to know the defects and dangers of the most commonly followed diets in America, read Part I, Chapter Two.

If you want to find out how recent history gave us the clues to unravelling the mystery of cancer, read Part II, Chapter Nine.

Read Part III to learn which foods you should avoid or eat to prevent cancer, and how to organize them into a balanced, attractive, and appetizing menu for lifelong nutrition.

If you want to learn about the scientific evidence behind the beta-carotene diet, read Part IV.

Now you know what this book is about. Let's look next at what it is *not*.

What This Book Is *Not*

- This is not an ordinary diet book, weight loss book, or nutrition manual, another one of which emerges every three months or so like a phoenix from the ashes of last year's remaindered list, repackaged and newly titled, only to subside after the public frenzy has run its course. If any such volume held the elusive key to eating well, losing weight, remaining slender, staying healthy, universal validity and perpetual use, and all the other promises explicit or implied, it would truly be the last diet book ever written.

  Many published diet books are potentially dangerous, even bizarre, in the peculiar foodstuffs they earnestly advocate. Most are merely last year's model recycled with a new paint job and a bit of buff and polish but no less flawed, with temporary unsustainable weight loss achieved at the cost of metabolic derangement.
- We will *not* count calories.
- We will *not* count grams of carbohydrates or anything else. Grams and calories—the quantity and energy content of foods—will be discussed, then forgotten, in favor of their automatic inclusion, correctly balanced in the beta-carotene diet structure.

- Exercise, aerobics, isometrics, jogging, calisthenics, and marathons are not relevant to what you will read in this book. At present there is no evidence that exercise bears any relationship, positive or negative, to cancer. That is not to say that I am advising you to remain slumped in an easy chair. As for weight loss, it takes half an hour of walking to burn off 100 calories, the number in two thin slices of bread. Exercise does bear a beneficial relationship to blood pressure, diabetes, and heart disease—more about that later.
- There will be no scales for daily weigh-ins, calipers to measure skinfolds, or tape measures to encompass your girth after every meal. In short, the emphasis is off anxiety (which may act as a trigger for some cancers), off adding another stress to the ones you already have, off a list of don'ts, and onto a simple formula for good health.
- There will be no complex food lists to refer to nor computations requiring a computer terminal or portable calculator to perform.
- You will not find food fads or nutritional fantasies here. Nutrition is a science.
- This book is *not* another cookie-cutter diet manual.

If you insist on miracles, I believe you will find more of a down-to-earth miracle (if that's not a contradiction), or at least an exciting new breakthrough, in the pages of this book than on a shelf full of last year's diet bestsellers.

That's enough of what this book is *not*. In the next chapter you'll find out what other diet books are not, even if some of them have camouflaged their metabolic mayhem with scientific sounding language, precise lists of minutiae, and mandatory diet rituals.

TWO

NEW YORK
vs.
CALIFORNIA

Neurologists, medical specialists in the diagnosis of disorders of the nervous system, are always talking about whether patients are "oriented times three." It's the first step in their evaluation of a patient's cerebral function: the ability to think clearly. Before checking your muscle function, touch perception, and reflexes, the neurologist will ask you to identify time, place, and person: the date, where you are, and who you are.

This primary location of the self in different dimensions seems to be operating subconsciously when diet doctors (and nondoctors) are naming their new diet books.

Some diet books focus on *time: The 9-Day Wonder Diet, The Easy 24-Hour Diet, The 30 Minutes a Week Diet, The 14-Day Shape-Up Program, The Over-35 Diet,* and *The Thin Forever Diet.*

Most *time* diets seem not to have withstood the test of time. Few readers will remember many of them. *Person* and *place* diets have been more popular recently.

The Atkins and Pritikin diets are the best known *person* diets of the last decade, while the Scarsdale and Beverly Hills diets take first place in the *place* diet category. More details about these leading diet approaches will follow.

You can find other categories if you look at the diet names listed in *Rating the Diets,* a sober compilation and commentary on the diet maze by Theodore Berland and the Editors of *Consumer Guide* (Signet Books, 1979).

You can choose from *The Boston Police Diet* or, if you like high places, *The Astronaut Diet* or, if you're political, *The U.S. Senate Diet*. If you're into royalty there's always *The Royal Swedish Diet*.

Diets that dare to mention food in their names give you a choice of *The Wine Diet, The Yogurt Diet, The Candy Diet, The Grapefruit Diet*, and even *The Drinking Man's Diet*.

There are diets that promise you can eat anything and everything as much as you want and still lose weight in health and safety. How do they do it? It defies all the laws of chemistry and biology (and gravity, too, for that matter).

Most diet books emphasize weight loss—weight loss without difficulty, weight loss without much valid scientific attention to health and safety.

Do people lose weight on such diets? Very often they do but, in most cases, temporarily. Many of the diet formulas ignore human metabolism, provoking unpleasant symptoms and dangerous biochemical abnormalities.

The other serious objection physicians and nutritionists raise is that most of the diets were never meant to be followed very long, without dire effects on the dieter. Without nutritionally sound new eating habits and without a sense of the psychological, cultural, and family roots behind habitual overeating, the temporarily successful dieter is doomed to "balloon out" again and again.

Let's take a look now at the Big Four diets of recent years and see how they stack up against the no-nonsense criteria of nutritional science. From their flaws and fallacies we will begin to shape The Ultimate Good Diet.

The Atkins Diet (*Dr. Atkins' Diet Revolution*, Bantam Books, 1973) is high in fat, low in carbohydrate. Without carbohydrate to burn for energy, the body breaks down stored fat instead. The fat breakdown produces ketones; carbohydrate shortage induces water loss. You will lose weight following this diet.

Why then did the Atkins diet provoke such controversy and criticism from well regarded medical sources?

1. Diets high in animal (saturated) fat and cholesterol are established as one of the three major risk factors for heart attack in particular and for cardiovascular disease in general.

8

2. Ketosis alters body chemistry. Our cells function best in a narrow range of the acid–alkali scale. Ketone bodies build up in the blood from fat breakdown faster than the body can excrete the ketones, increasing the acidity of body fluids and tissues. Altering our "internal environment" (as it was so neatly termed by Claude Bernard, a famous French physiologist who predated Atkins by more than a century) is very damaging, especially to diabetics, during pregnancy to the unborn child, and in gout and kidney disorders.

3. High-fat, ketogenic diets are unpleasant, leading to diarrhea, dehydration, foul breath, fatigue, and weakness.

The low fat, low calorie Pritikin Diet (*The Pritikin Program for Diet & Exercise*, Bantam Books, 1980) requires the almost constant consumption of large quantities of vegetables. This provides very little fat or free sugar, sparse calories, and not much protein. Walking several miles a day is part of the plan. You will lose weight following this diet.

But realistically, what are the inherent defects of such a diet? How many of us can stay on a diet that would make only a rabbit happy, or put in the daily mileage of a gazelle on an African plain? Even if you are that rare hybrid human with a rabbit's appetite and a gazelle's legs, the diet may cause gas and diarrhea and provide insufficient fat for flavor or sense of satisfaction after eating and inadequate protein for body repair and maintenance or for the needs of adolescents or pregnant women. Pritikin in his revised diet added cottage cheese to the vegetable regimen in an attempt to remedy at least the insufficient protein of his diet.

In the high protein Scarsdale Diet (*The Complete Scarsdale Medical Diet*, Bantam Books, 1980) the dieter is encouraged to consume large but unspecified amounts of protein. The diet attempts to limit fat, especially of animal origin (saturated), and provides moderate carbohydrate. Menus are rigidly prescribed as to specific foods at the same time that quantities are left to the reader's discretion.

If you follow this diet you will lose weight, probably because your total caloric consumption will be less than usual as a result of limiting fats and proscribing between-meal and late-night snacking, alcohol, and sweets.

But the diet is not intended for permanent eating habit modification, a cardinal rule of correct nutrition. After temporary dieting, weight tends to be regained. Foods high in protein are usually high in undesirable cholesterol and sometimes also in fats. Protein break-

9

down products must be excreted by the kidneys. People with less than normal kidney function, or liver disease or gout, should limit protein intake. Because the diet induces rapid fat breakdown with ketone accumulation, it should be avoided by diabetics. Bad breath and fatigue are also side effects.

In an article in the *Journal of the American Medical Association* (Gabe B. Mirkin, M.D., University of Maryland, and Ronald N. Shore, M.D., The Johns Hopkins University School of Medicine, November 13, 1981), the Beverly Hills Diet (Berkley Books, 1982) is described as ". . . perhaps the worst entry in the diet-fad derby. The diet's major tenets fly in the face of all established medical knowledge about nutrition." The authors state: "In our opinion, the Beverly Hills diet preaches nutritional nonsense." As they point out, there are no shortcuts, revolutionary miracle breakthroughs, or easy routes to weight loss. To lose excess fat you must eat fewer calories than your body consumes for its energy requirements—there is no other way. Faddish, unscientific, and dangerous diet books will continue to sell well until the modern alchemist's dream of just melting excess weight away is abandoned.

You begin the Beverly Hills diet by eating only fruit for the first eleven days, a diet that can produce severe diarrhea, unpleasant enough in itself, but that can lead to a dangerous drop in blood pressure to shock levels, due to decreased blood volume. You also risk potassium deficiency with generalized muscle weakness and potentially dangerous heart rhythms. During the first six weeks on the diet there is so little protein that massive hair loss may result. The Beverly Hills diet is based on scientifically invalid theories totally at odds with the basic facts about human digestion, enzymes, and nutrition.

The *Journal of the AMA* article lists numerous scientific errors in the Beverly Hills diet book. Critical review focuses on the three main concepts of the book:

1. That only undigested food will accumulate and become fat in the body, while fully digested food will not produce weight gain.
2. That most enzyme systems cannot function effectively at the same time in the body.
3. That the enzymes present in fruits are effective in making hard-to-digest foods less fattening.

It does not take an advanced degree in nutritional science to separate fallacy from fact about the Beverly Hills diet. Undigested food cannot be fattening because it will not be absorbed by the body from the gastrointestinal tract and will be excreted in the stool. It can be, and has been, easily demonstrated that numerous enzymes work simultaneously in the process of digestion, first in the mouth, then in the stomach, and last in the small intestine. Almost all foods contain varying proportions of the three basic food components, carbohydrate, fat, and protein, each of which calls for a different enzyme system to break down the large molecular structures that occur naturally in food into fragments small enough to be absorbed through the wall of the intestine. The digestive enzymes produced by the body should not be confused with enzymes naturally present in foods. Food enzymes are themselves proteins, so that none of them make it through the stomach intact without being digested (broken down) by stomach enzymes into amino acids, which are inert from a digestive point of view.

OK, then, what *is* a good diet?

THREE

WHAT
IS A GOOD
DIET?

First, what is a *diet?* Diet means different things, sometimes confusing. Your diet is what you ordinarily eat and drink. A diet implies a departure from your habitual fare, a limitation or selection of the kinds or amounts of foods consumed. It may be prescribed by a doctor—usually a long-term change if it is—for example, salt restriction for high blood pressure or fat-free foods for gallbladder disease. Self-prescribed diets are usually short-term ventures if weight reduction is the goal. One purpose of this book is to alter mass eating habits in the direction dictated by the Unified Concept of Cancer and Cardiovascular Disease Prevention with Weight Control.

Impossible, you're thinking, we'll never get Americans to give up their charcoal-broiled steaks, butter, and cheese. But we're already doing it, as you will learn in Chapter Six. Dietary modification, not total abstinence from the gustatory goodies we learned to love in childhood, is our goal. And successive generations not brought up on the high risk cancer and heart disease diets we are accustomed to eating and conditioned to believe healthy, will not have to recondition their palates.

- A good diet must be a comfortable lifetime eating pattern.
- To understand what a good diet is we need to have a clearcut understanding of the meaning of the component parts: first, protein, carbohydrate, and fat.

Protein

Proteins are biochemical compounds consisting of chains of amino acids, which in turn consist of carbon, oxygen, hydrogen, and nitrogen, and occasionally other elements. Proteins are the building blocks of plant and animal structure, the major constituent of cell protoplasm, and the source of our enzymes and genes. Albumin and globulin are kinds of human protein.

Carbohydrates

Carbohydrates are organic compounds composed of various arrangements and chains of carbon, oxygen, and hydrogen. Sugar, starch, and cellulose are carbohydrates. They are our most direct energy source.

Fat

Fats are oily substances, white or yellow tissue, which provide a reserve energy supply. In biologic terms they are organic compounds, in the language of biochemists, they are known as glyceryl esters of fatty acids.

Fats are saturated or unsaturated. Unsaturated fats can be further divided into monounsaturated and polyunsaturated. Saturation is a chemical distinction relating to whether or not a compound can combine readily with other chemical substances. Biologically it is important because saturated fats, the type found in fats of animal origin (and in a few plant foods, such as coconuts), appear to be the culprit in arteriosclerosis (hardening of the arteries)—coronary heart disease. Monounsaturated fat is found in substances such as olive oil, and polyunsaturated fat is found in corn oil. Without getting ahead of ourselves at this point, I will say that all three forms of fat, particularly saturated fat, are related to cancer.

Two other words we use in talking about food are gram and calorie.

Gram

A gram is a very small measure of weight in the metric system, the system in general use throughout Europe and used in America for scientific purposes. There are about 500 grams in a pound (454 grams to the pound, to be more exact).

Calorie

A calorie is a measure of energy. It is defined, when we are talking about the caloric content of foods, as the amount of heat energy available in the food sufficient to raise the temperature of one thousand grams of water (equal to about one quart of water) by one degree centigrade.

There are wide variations, but 2,000 calories per day for women and 2,500 calories per day for men represent typical daily caloric needs for healthy active adults.

Cholesterol

Cholesterol is a crystalline fatty alcohol so important in human biology that I will list its chemical formula here—$C_{27}H_{45}OH$. Cholesterol is a fatty substance found in association with animal fat.

Cholesterol, major villain of the twentieth-century cardiovascular epidemic, is an important precursor—a building block—in the synthesis of adrenal, ovarian, and testicular hormones (cortisone, estrogen and progesterone, and testosterone). Cholesterol, however, can be synthesized by our bodies from what are called *acetate radicals*. So cholesterol derived from food sources may not be essential.

Salt

Ordinary table salt is a compound, the chemical combination of two elements, sodium and chloride. It is the sodium fraction of common table salt that appears to be the villain in many forms of hypertension and the fluid retention associated with heart, liver, and kidney disease. Sodium is a component of sodium bicarbonate, $NaHCO_3$, also known as common baking soda used in cooking as a leavening agent to raise dough by releasing carbon dioxide. Sodium is also part of monosodium glutamate, a flavor enhancer often used in Chinese cooking. Ordinary salt is, of course, also used in the preparation of salt-cured foods. Sodium from any source may be a problem for people with cardiovascular disease.

Sugar

Sugar is a carbohydrate but, like fat, consists of different subgroups, some of which are better than others when included in the diet. Free sugar or simple sugar, such as glucose, sucrose, or fructose, tastes sweet. The table sugar that you find in the sugar bowl is a simple sugar, a molecule that needs little digestion. It is rapidly absorbed from the digestive tract, producing a swift rise in blood sugar levels and problems for patients with diabetes, whose insulin response mechanisms are unable to cope with such quick shifts in blood sugar levels.

Complex carbohydrates, such as cellulose and starches, consist of long molecular chains of sugarlike fragments. Because of their prolonged digestion (breakdown within the digestive tract), they provide a slower, smoother shift in blood sugar levels, an advantage to nondiabetics as well as diabetics by avoiding abrupt swings in blood sugar, an important factor in vascular (blood vessel) disease.

Fiber

Dietary fiber includes crude fiber (cellulose, hemicellulose, and lignin), the undigestible remnants of the plant cell structure, plus pectins, gums and indigestible animal tissues. Fiber is not absorbed into the body, but by accelerating food transit time through the gastrointestinal tract, it decreases the duration of contact between carcinogens in food or bile acids and the bowel wall. Many observers feel that it is of value in decreasing bowel cancer. Whole grains, fruits, and vegetables are good sources. About 30 grams of dietary fiber per day (equivalent to 5 to 6 grams of crude fiber) is ample.

Food Groups

Grains, fruits, vegetables, and dairy and meat products constitute the four main food groups. In Chapter 13 we will look at some subdivisions and examples of each group and how they provide the protein, carbohydrate, and fat in our diet.

Vitamins

Vitamins act as enzymes. The human body itself produces most of the enzymes it needs. The relatively small number of enzymes our bodies are unable to synthesize are what we call *vitamins*, which must be obtained from food. Chemically, enzymes are known as *catalysts*. Many chemical reactions will proceed slowly without the presence of a catalyst or enzyme, but even minute amounts of the catalyst will greatly accelerate the rate of a reaction. The catalysts or enzymes or vitamins are not ordinarily stored by the human body. They are not synthesized, so they must be consumed frequently, preferably daily, for optimum health. Deficiency states, that is, clinically recognizable symptoms or groups of symptoms called syndromes, begin to appear after weeks or months of vitamin deprivation [diseases such as pellagra (niacin, a B vitamin), beriberi (thiamine, Vitamin B_1) or scurvy (Vitamin C)]. Not all animal species have identical vitamin needs. Dogs, for example, are able to synthesize Vitamin C. There is nothing mysterious or magical about vitamins. They have been blessed by an imaginative name derived from the Latin root meaning life, and have benefitted from a good press and aggressive advertising. But they are simply chemical substances that facilitate everyday biochemical reactions in our bodies. Yes, it *is* controversial, but consuming more than the tiny quantities needed is useless. Excessive doses of vitamins are not absorbed or are rapidly excreted from the body. It is toxic to take chronic overdoses of some vitamins.

Vitamin A (retinol): Fat soluble. Related to vision, skin and membrane integrity. Found in liver, butter, egg yolk, cheese, tomato, and many vegetables. Precursor: carotene. Toxicity: enlarged spleen and liver, bone marrow depression, bone and hair changes.

Vitamin B Complex: Water soluble. Involved in many enzyme

16

systems. Found in green, leafy vegetables, milk, lean meat, and grains. Vitamin B_1 (thiamine) is required by the heart and nerves. Deficiency state: beriberi. Vitamin B_2 (riboflavin) deficiency affects the eyes, mouth, and skin. Niacin (nicotinic acid) affects the mouth, skin, intestinal tract, and brain. Deficiency state: pellagra. Other B vitamins, Vitamin B_{12}, Folic Acid, and Vitamin B_6 (pyridoxine), affect blood formation or nerve function.

Vitamin C (ascorbic acid): Water soluble. Found in citrus fruits and tomatoes and in many raw vegetables. Deficiency state: scurvy, manifested by hair loss, skin changes, hemorrhaging, loss of teeth, and bone fractures. High doses of Vitamin C can damage growing bones, or provoke gout or kidney stones, and sickle crisis in susceptible persons.

Vitamin D (calciferol, Vitamin D_2 or activated 7–dehydrocholesterol, Vitamin D_3): Fat soluble. Found in fish, liver, butter, egg yolk, added to milk, and produced by the body on exposure to sunlight. Deficiency state: rickets, a disorder of bone formation. Toxicity: induces high blood calcium, causing gastrointestinal and urinary symptoms, headache, weakness, and loss of appetite.

Vitamin E (alpha-tocopherol): Fat soluble. Found in wheat, cereals, egg yolk, beef liver. Metabolic changes due to a deficiency of Vitamin E have been hard to identify with certainty.

Vitamin K: Fat soluble. Deficiency causes bleeding due to low prothrombin blood levels.

Minerals

Minerals are elements, such as iron, copper, zinc, and selenium, some of which play important roles in normal human physiology. Just as for vitamins, the amounts needed are very small and are comfortably found in anything resembling a normal diet. There are deficiency and toxicity states, too. Iron deficiency can produce anemia, but excessive iron can produce a potentially much graver disease as a result of chronic deposition of iron in the liver and pancreas.

Almost one out of two Americans take vitamins and minerals, at a total cost of two to three billion dollars per year. Very few benefit.

TABLE I

Recommended Daily Requirements

	Vitamins
Vitamin A	5,000 IU (International Units)
Vitamin D	400 IU
Vitamin E	30 IU
Vitamin K	70–140 μg (micrograms)
Vitamin B$_1$	1.5 mg (milligrams)
Vitamin B$_2$	1.7 mg
Niacin	20.0 mg
Vitamin B$_6$	2.0 mg
Vitamin B$_{12}$	6.0 μg
Folacin	0.4 mg
Biotin	0.3 mg
Pantothenic Acid	10.0 mg
Vitamin C	60.0 mg
	Minerals
Calcium	800 mg
Phosphorus	800 mg
Magnesium	300–350 mg
Iron	10–18 mg
Zinc	15 mg
Iodine	150 μg
Copper	2.0–3.0 mg
Manganese	2.5–5.0 mg
Fluoride	1.5–4.0 mg
Chromium	0.05–0.2 mg
Selenium	0.05–0.2 mg
Molybdenum	0.15–0.5 mg
	Electrolytes (salts)
Sodium	1,100–3,300 mg
Potassium	1,875–5,625 mg
Chloride	1,700–5,100 mg

TABLE II

Food	Diet Goal	
Carbohydrate	58% of total calories	
Complex (starches, etc.)	48%	
Simple (sugars)	10%	
Fat	30% of total calories	
Saturated	10%	
Monounsaturated	10%	
Polyunsaturated	10%	
Protein	12% of total calories	
Cholesterol	less than 300 mg per day	
Salt	less than 5 gms per day	

Example: 2,000-Calorie Diet

	Percent	Grams	Calories
Carbohydrate	58	315	1,260
Fat	30	66⅔	600
Protein	12	60	240
		Total	2,000

How Much Protein, Carbohydrate, and Fat Do We Need?

Nutritionists have come up with the following daily minimum needs for protein, carbohydrate, and fat.

Protein

Fifty grams are adequate—fewer are not enough for normal repair and maintenance of body tissues. Much higher amounts are not beneficial and in fact may be dangerous for people with kidney and liver disease. High protein intake is also linked to increased fat intake, because the two so often are found together, especially in foods of animal origin. Sixty to eighty grams of protein per day, although not damaging to a normal adult, are not really necessary. Children require proportionately more protein than is adequate for the repair and maintenance needs of adults. Protein in excess of body needs enters the metabolic pool of nutrients, undergoes conversion, and emerges as fat or sugar.

Carbohydrate

Minimum needs are set at 60 grams per day. With lower amounts, fat is broken down instead of carbohydrate to provide energy, which may lead to ketosis, an abnormal acid state that disturbs cell metabolism and body biochemistry. Much higher amounts of carbohydrate may be needed to meet energy needs, carbohydrate being the primary source of energy, with amounts up to several hundred grams per day necessary for people engaged in strenuous physical activity.

Fat

Fats have traditionally provided 40 percent or even more of the total calories in the customary American diet. Recent studies have shown that this should be reduced to 30 percent of total calories or possibly lower—split three ways into saturated, monounsaturated, and polyunsaturated—because of the impact of fat not only on the cardiovascular system, but on the genesis of cancer. Fats contain 9 calories per gram, carbohydrates and protein only 4 calories per gram. To put that in perspective, in customary American weights and measures, one ounce—1/16 of a pound—of carbohydrate or protein has 113 calories, while one ounce of fat has 255 calories.

Fat supposedly increases the palatability of foods. Such taste preference most likely is conditioned rather than intrinsic, so we can unlearn it. Conditioning children's food tastes is advisable. Fats do play a nutritional role in providing a vehicle for the fat soluble vitamins A and D.

Food Groups
and the Diet

From the food groups of grains, fruits, vegetables, and dairy and meat products, our task is to select foods that will have appropriate amounts of protein, carbohydrate, fat, vitamins, minerals, and fiber. The diet must be palatable, the foods available, and long-term acceptance by most people reasonably certain. It must be a diet that can be adapted to the growth needs of the young, the special needs of pregnancy, sedentary or physically active adults, and the elderly. It must be adaptable to the medical problems of persons with diabetes, gout, kidney and liver disease, and cardiovascular ailments.

Goals

We are concerned not just with weight loss or gain, but with health maintenance and improvement. Most diet books focus on weight loss in its cosmetic or psychological aspects. Often risky to health, rapid weight loss is as a rule brief in duration and unsustainable. Many of us accept bizarre dietary gyrations because they are in print. Weight loss achieved at the cost of metabolic derangement will not endure. Only a permanent new eating habit in which health is a goal at least as important as weight loss will produce permanent benefits.

For many decades, in our culture at least, thin, slender, or trim has seemed more desirable than fat, gross, or obese. Whether a cultural imperative or cosmetic preference, thin seems to correlate with youth, beauty, and vigor and overweight with sloth, decadence, and apathy. Perhaps the preference for thin has been more than skin deep, a psychological throwback to the natural state of primitive man. The emerging evidence of a definite relationship between low body weight, good health, relative immunity to cardiovascular disorders, and protection against cancer should lend fervor to your pursuit of a lean body and knowledgeable food choices.

To consume unconventional diets without scientific proof of validity, to accept claims of promoting good health or treating specific disease conditions, and to use food supplements or excessive amounts of vitamins is simply to squander a great opportunity for good health and long life.

FOUR

NOTES, NUMBERS, AND THOUGHTS

The Old Water Trick

In the days when cattle herds were driven on foot to market instead of taking the train, there was a trick played by herdsmen on the packing company buyers, called *watering the stock*. For days before reaching the big markets in Omaha, Kansas City, and Chicago, the cattle were systematically deprived of water. Hours before reaching the slaughterhouses they were fed salt, then at last allowed to drink their fill from the nearest stream or river. The great beasts, dusty and dehydrated, thereby turned water at $0.00 per gallon into money at $4.98 per pound, or whatever the equivalent going price at the stockyards was then for meat on the hoof: hence the expression *watered stock*. This phrase was taken over and applied to the great stock market swindles of the 1870s, when the financial robber barons of Wall Street were making fortunes by inflating and deflating stock prices by rumors, ploys, and manipulations.

The old water trick is still with us today! The substantial weight loss that occurs during the first few days of some highly touted quick weight loss diets consists almost entirely of water loss. During an absolute fast your real weight loss is 0.6–0.7 pounds per day. Any apparent weight loss beyond 0.7 pounds per day consists of fluid. The key relationship to remember between calories and pounds is that to lose one pound of genuine body weight requires a 3,500-calorie deficit, 3,500 fewer calories eaten than are needed by your body to maintain caloric equilibrium—calories consumed in food versus calories expended to meet basic energy requirements. If we take 2,500 calories as a typical daily caloric requirement for the average adult male (2,000 calories for the average adult female), with zero food intake the man will lose 0.71 pounds and the woman 0.57 pounds per day. This, of course, is not a recommended diet scheme, but a man on such a fast will lose only approximately five pounds per week of true weight. Any diet promising more is tricking you with a metabolic doublecross by counting water loss. Overweight people do tend to have water retention, but after the initial rapid diuresis (water loss) progresses to relative dehydration, a state that is physiologically unsound and potentially dangerous, natural thirst and water consumption produce a Ping-Pong or pendulum effect on body fluid balance and weight.

We need a minimum of 600 cc of urine per day to excrete waste products of metabolism from the body. Keeping in mind that one liter of fluid measure is equal to 1000 cc and is virtually equivalent to one quart of liquid in our everyday measuring system, 600 cc equals just over one-half quart of fluid. An ordinary teaspoon, by the way, holds about 4 or 5 cc. Most people in normal health will actually excrete 1,000 to 1,500 cc of urine per day. That is easier on the kidneys, which do not have to work so hard to concentrate the same amount of waste material into a smaller volume of liquid. Many of us consume 2,000 cc of liquid per day in various forms, although that amount may vary considerably, depending on personal preference, climate, and physical activity. The difference between the amount of liquid consumed and urine excreted is made up by perspiration, exhaled water vapor, and the moisture contained in stool.

Each liter of urine (1,000 cc) weighs one kilogram (1,000 grams) or, in our equivalent daily measuring system, each quart weighs about 2.2 pounds. Overweight people retain water, particularly if excessive salt intake has been habitual. Some water is probably held in physical or chemical combination with fat deposits, some in the blood vessel system, and the rest in the cells and intercellular spaces. A heavy diuresis begins when salt intake drops, thus requiring less liquid to hold the salt in solution. Rapid fat breakdown in low-carbohydrate diets frees additional water. Urine outflow under such circumstances may triple or quadruple from, say, 1,000 to 3,000—

4,000 cc per day. With each 1,000 cc or liter weighing 2.2 pounds, a weight loss, almost entirely of water, up to 5 pounds or more in a single day will thrill the obese patient, particularly if he or she has been encouraged to consume palate- and gut-satisfying quantities of protein and fat-filled foods at the same time. Psychological needs for satiation have been met and have been rewarded with an extraordinary loss of weight in one or two days. No wonder such diets make instant converts with a nationwide popularity that spreads as fast as delivery trucks can carry the printed word. Aside from the metabolic chaos and derangement to the internal milieu as dehydration sets in and thirst responds, never again is that initial flush of dramatic weight loss recaptured. Ecstasy turns ultimately to disappointment, or boredom with the diet leads to relapsing into previous eating habits. Whatever real weight might have been lost, not to mention the temporary wringing out of the water retained in fatty tissues, is then regained.

Drugs

I will not spend much time talking about various drugs that have been used from time to time to induce weight loss. Their use is condemned without exception and without question. At the very least they are not conducive to developing eating habits consistent with any rational approach to balanced nutrition. At their worst they are extremely dangerous. Amphetamines, which have been marketed under a wide variety of brand names, and the related drugs ordinarily used as nasal decongestants, such as phenylpropanolamine, may raise pulse rate and blood pressure to dangerous levels. The use of thyroid medication to accelerate body metabolism, or the heart drug digitalis in an effort to increase kidney blood flow and induce diuresis, are about as dangerous as racing your car blindfolded. Laxatives to provoke rapid transit of food through the intestines, or methylcellulose to create a sense of bulk in the stomach, have never worked well.

Obesity Surgery

Surgical procedures to short-circuit the stomach or intestines in patients 100 pounds overweight or more provoke mind boggling metabolic disorders, disastrous symptoms of gastrointestinal malfunction, and a high mortality rate.

Tobacco

Smoking as an appetite suppressant is probably the worst possible approach to weight loss.

Exercise

Exercising, although relaxing and possibly beneficial to the cardiovascular system, unfortunately consumes relatively few calories compared to controlling your diet. It takes 2 minutes to eat 2 thin slices of bread (100 calories) and a half-hour's walk to burn them off. One half hour of vigorous tennis takes only a donut and a soft drink to even the score (200 to 250 calories).

The Calorie-Pound Equation

Keep in mind the figure of 3,500 calories, the deficit below energy requirements to equal one pound of genuine weight loss. To lose weight, reasonable nutritionists advise dropping your caloric intake by 500 to 1,000 calories per day below the 2,000 to 2,500 needed by women and men for calorie input and energy output balance. A 500 calorie per day deficit will result in a one pound per week weight loss, and a 1,000 calorie per day deficit, in a two pound per week weight loss. Faced with taking off 20 to 30 pounds or more, you may be dismayed by the turtle's pace of one pound per week. But within a few months the desired weight will be reached, without sacrificing the necessary daily balance of 50 grams of protein, at least 60 grams of carbohydrate, and not more than 30 percent of total calories derived from fat (10 percent saturated, 10 percent monounsaturated, and 10 percent polyunsaturated).

To calculate the number of calories you need per day to maintain your present weight, a well-known rule of thumb is to multiply your weight by 15. That will give you a close approximation of your steady-state energy needs expressed in calories. For example, a 166 pound man multiplying his weight by 15 will come up with a daily caloric need of about 2,500 calories. A 133 pound woman multiplying her weight by 15 will find she needs about 2,000 calories a day to maintain her weight. A caloric intake greater on the average each day than those figures will lead to gradual weight gain; a caloric intake of a lower amount as a daily average will cause weight loss.

Diets with fewer than 1,000 to 1,200 calories are ill advised, leading as they do to fatigue and weakness and providing inadequate quantities of nutrients.

FIVE

ANCIENT MAN

For two million years man and his historical predecessors lived as hunters and gatherers of wild plants. Only about 10,000 years ago did man begin to plant, cultivate, and harvest. With the more rooted existence of planting and tending crops in a fixed location, the migrant or nomadic style was eventually replaced by a village existence. As a result of the cultivation of grain crops and development of the farm village, the domestication of sheep and goats from their wild antecedents became practical. It may have begun as early as 9200 BC in parts of what is now the Middle East or Southwest Asia. Thousands of years afterward the domestication of wild bovines followed, leading to the development of cattle herding, somewhere around the year 4000 B.C. The use of cattle for meat probably preceded their use for providing milk, which probably happened sometime between 3000 and 4000 B.C. Pigs and then poultry were probably domesticated around that time as well. The increased dependence on livestock for meat and milk, and the harvesting of grain crops, together constituted a profound change in the diet of man, compared to the leaner diet provided by wild berries and nuts, fruits and green plants, and the sporadic lean meat of wild animals caught by hunters. The farm revolution resulted in a food structure high in starches, and in animal fats derived from the sedentary cow and pig, as well as the fat content of dairy products and eggs. Although the change occupied 5,000 years in social history, it was barely a single moment on our genetic clocks. Even now, 7,000 years since man settled down to tend flocks and harvest crops, we still have the genetic apparatus of the hunter and the wild berry gatherer. Over tens of thousands of years, man evolved into a creature fit to survive in the wilderness. Little wonder, then, that our genes have not been able to adapt at the same speed in which we have manipulated the environment around us and altered the pattern of foods we consume. In such a context it becomes less mysterious that the changes around and within us may account for the twin epidemics of cardiovascular disease and cancer. It is a question we shall pursue.

There are some clues as well in anthropology:

- In the longevity of Russian peasants in the Ural Mountains.
- In the rarity of breast cancer in Japanese and Hawaiians until they emigrate to the continental United States.
- In the difference in breast cancer incidence between European and North African Jews until they emigrate to Israel.
- In the high incidence of liver cancer in the Chinese, esophageal cancer in the Finns, primary liver cancer in parts of Africa, and Burkitt's lymphoma in children living near the Sahara Desert.

From such inquiry, threads are emerging that suggest connections and causes.

SIX

THE ULTIMATE GOOD DIET

Most diets of the last two decades have been flawed in different ways:

- Weight loss at any metabolic cost.
- Health motivated but without regard to palatability or practicality.
- Required computer age technology to keep track of grams or calories.
- Based on fanciful or unsound theorizing.
- Not good on weekends, holidays, or for a lifetime.

The ultimate good diet for these final two decades of the century must score 7 out of 7 on the Ultimate Diet Scale if it is to get us all safely to the year 2,000 and beyond.

The Ultimate Diet Test

1. *Cost and availability:* If researchers in the obscure lab outside Moscow should emerge next May Day with the assertion that a high caviar diet was responsible for the remarkable longevity of people in the Ural Mountains region of the Soviet Union, it would do most of us very little good, the world supply of caviar being extremely limited.

2. *Palatability and practicality:* Only eskimos would rejoice over the unexpected news that whale blubber conveys magical health

benefits. Most of us would still prefer to take our chances with cheeseburgers and milkshakes. Ultimate foods must also be easy to transport to the point of consumption, store well, be easy to prepare, and conform to culturally acceptable patterns of eating. Aside from newborns, not many of us will set the alarm clock to get up at 3 A.M. to consume a middle-of-the-night feeding.

3. *Simplicity, flexibility, and fun:* Nature seems to have built certain pleasurable inducements into preservation of the species and the self. If sex and eating were merely duties, we would never have made it out of the Neanderthal stage. Your daily fare must be fun. Complexity of preparation or monotony of consumption will quickly doom any diet.

4. *Acceptability:* Once established as a national norm, "being on a diet" should be forgotten.

5. *Permanence:* Foods should be readily available at all times.

6. *Conformity to scientific health principles:* Foods should result in a balanced diet.

7. *Suitability for subgroups of the population:* Children and the elderly; the sedentary or physically active; male or female; pregnant women; and people with a variety of diseases, such as hypertension, diabetes, or diverticulosis must be able to adapt the basic diet to their particular needs.

Is it possible to create mass shifts in population behavior? Certainly. Look around the world. Dietary practices vary enormously in different cultures. There is nothing sacrosanct in or intrinsic to current American or Western European food preferences. Southeast Asians do very well on rice, grain and fish. Some Africans subsist mostly on meats, others solely on vegetables, and some Pacific islanders, on tropical fruits. In large measure chance, availability, climate, and childhood conditioning determine our tastes.

We are not talking about dramatic dietary twists and turns or convolutions. Rutabaga roots or sautéed eel would turn most of us away. Fortunately modest shifts in diet will suffice.

There is an excellent evidence that people do respond enthusiastically to concerted public health campaigns. During the

1970s the death rate from cardiovascular disease decreased 25 percent from the expected levels (a quarter of a million lives saved each year). Medical authorities attribute the decrease to the promotion of changes in lifestyle: weight loss, decreased animal fat, sugar, and salt in the diet, attention to blood pressure, increased exercise, and less cigarette smoking. The advertising and marketing media skills of Madison Avenue can serve us well in the public health sphere. The decade of the 1970s will be remembered as the beginning of the prevention of heart disease. Perhaps the 1980s will be hailed for the prevention of cancer.

An overview of health progress in the twentieth century focuses on three phases:

1. *Public health:* control of infection through improvements in purity of the water and food supply, immunization, and antibiotics.
2. *Technology:* improvements in diagnosis and treatment, a mushrooming drug industry, and the dawn of genetic engineering and immunology.
3. *The lifestyle revolution:* the key to controlling heart disease and cancer.

Diet plays a major role in the prevention of heart disease and cancer, but is there a "Catch-22" here? Will a cardiac protective diet be incompatible with cancer prevention, and vice versa?

Happily, the answer is no. The Unified Concept of Cancer and Cardiovascular Disease Prevention depends on a curious compatibility, an overlap between the two diets. The same foods play one role in the prevention of heart disease and another in the prevention of cancer. I suggest that there is a connection, an evolutionary link with the historical genetic makeup of the human race, rooted in the habits, circumstances, and preferences of primitive man.

The reader in this next to the last decade of the twentieth century is familiar with the risk factors for coronary heart disease:

1. A diet high in saturated (animal) fat and cholesterol and low in fiber.
2. Obesity.
3. Diabetes, a disorder of sugar metabolism.
4. Hypertension (high blood pressure).
5. Lack of exercise.
6. Cigarette smoking.

Many of the factors, particularly the dietary ones, play a major role in carcinogenesis—the inception of cancer. There is a set of foods that can dramatically increase your probability of contracting cancer and, just as dramatically, another set of foods that can protect you against cancer.

With 50 percent of all deaths in the United States caused by cardiovascular disease and 20 to 25 percent by cancer, the outlook is exciting: A long, healthy, productive lifespan is coming within our reach.

WHAT IS CANCER?

SEVEN

UNDERSTANDING CANCER

What is cancer? What causes it? Why do some people get cancer and others not? Can we prevent it? Why does cancer occur more in certain organs than others? Why are there differences in the cancers of men and women? How does age affect vulnerability to cancer? Why are there ethnic and racial differences in cancer incidence? Is it genetic? What is the role of the environment?

Just a few decades ago cancer was viewed as maverick tissue, which had inexplicably arisen and turned against its own body. Cause, prevention, and cure were speculative; fear and the outcome, a foregone conclusion—that is, until 40 years ago. In 1941 researcher Isaac Berenblum, M.D., using chemicals (benzpyrene and croton resin) painted on mouse skin showed that the development of a cancer was an understandable three-part process: initiation, latency, and promotion.

Initiation involves a basic change in the genes of affected cells—a mutation—an alteration of the correct composition of DNA (deoxyribonucleic acid), the chemical code or program of all life forms.

A mutated cell need not develop into a clinical cancer. A very long—even lifelong—period of dormancy follows mutation: the latency period.

A separate process, promotion, must occur for the mutated cells to begin to reproduce their faulty cellular geography. A mutation

35

having once occurred cannot be reversed, but promotion, a long, slow process, can be prevented or, once begun, halted and latency restored. The independent process of promotion can be provoked by the same agent that caused the initial mutant change or by a different agent.

Understanding of the genetic code within our cells has leapfrogged over the biological sciences in a startling number of directions and has given us a unified grasp of what once seemed to be so unrelated. The long, coiled strands of amino acids (protein building blocks) in DNA contain the hereditary code for each form of life that is passed from generation to generation. DNA is also the blueprint for the structure and function of each living organism, the master code governing the development and reproduction of every cell in the body. It is fascinating that virus particles are also small packets of DNA. The growing science of immunology deals with the way our DNA mobilizes antibodies to cope with viruses. Immunology also studies diseases of the immune system itself (autoimmune diseases) characterized by antibody formation against the body's own cells. Cancer is just an aberration of DNA, against which the immune system mobilizes its defense mechanisms, destroying faulty DNA in the same way as any other substance foreign to the body. Cancer occurs if and when the immune mechanism is overwhelmed or rendered futile. Cancer is no longer the inexplicable nightmare it once was—its cause can be understood, prevention devised, and cure conceived.

Considering our billions of cells, length of life, frequency of cell division, and vast array of hostile environmental substances to which we are exposed, the occurrence of clinical cancer is a rare event.

Therefore, reproduction, structure and function, growth and development; immune responses to invaders from without or mutant genes from within; and cancer have a common origin in DNA. It is not too elusive for the mind to unravel and to rearrange for our benefit and protection.

Before closing our discussion of the general characteristics of cancer, it will be helpful to understand some definitions. There are three main classifications of cancer in people, depending on the tissue of origin:

1. *Carcinoma* arises in the tissues of functioning organs such as the lungs, stomach, colon, reproductive organs, and hormone producing glands.
2. *Sarcoma* occurs in connective tissues—bone and muscle.
3. *Lymphoma* is found in lymph nodes and bone marrow.

Different cancers have different patterns:

- Affect one sex more than the other (e.g., breast cancer in women).
- Affect different age groups (prostate cancer in older men).
- Affect different ethnic groups (liver cancer in Chinese or esophageal cancer in Finns).
- May be fast growing or slow growing (melanoma of the skin—fast; basal cell carcinoma of the skin—slow).
- Affect different occupations (lung cancer in asbestos workers).

A primary cancer means it has originated in that organ; a secondary or metastatic cancer has arisen elsewhere in the body and spread via the blood or lymphatic channels. Cancer may be locally invasive, spreading directly to adjacent organs. Cancers tend to have specific pathways of spread that they follow: stomach and colon to the liver, prostate to the vertebral bones, lung to the brain, breast to the ribs and pleura, and so on.

Although not likely to become household words, *oncogenes* and *transposons,* recent words that sound more like science fiction than science fact, are showing up in scientific publications more and more. The oncogene is a gene with malignant potential; the transposon acts as a genetic trigger.

The fact that cancer in general is more common in older age groups has led to some provocative and useful speculation. Are we seeing more cancer simply because people are living longer because of the improved control of infectious and cardiovascular diseases? Are new environmental factors in our industrial age responsible? Is decreased ability with age to repair faulty DNA a factor? Does the immune system in youth better recognize mutant DNA as foreign and act to expel it, a capacity that is lost with age? Is there truly an outer limit to the length of human life (some say 100 years, based on lab studies showing that human cells can reproduce no more than 50 times in tissue culture)?

EIGHT

CASE
HISTORIES

Melissa Sue Miller walked off the club court after a close match with her old friend and tennis rival, Jennie Potter. Melissa hesitated for a moment at her car door.

"You said you had something important to talk to me about," said Jennie.

Melissa's face clouded over. She was, at 35, attractive and happy.

"There is something," she began with hesitation. "I haven't even told Jerry about it." Jennie prepared herself. She had heard this preamble before, but the next sentence was never the same.

"For four months now," Melissa began again, "I've had this little thing. . . in the breast. I thought it would just go away. I've had cysts before, you know."

"Did you see Dr. Perry?" asked Jennie.

"No," said Melissa, "I've been afraid to. I thought I'd wait and ask you what to do."

"Well, if you're worried about it, why don't you see your doctor?"

"I suppose I should, but I'm really scared about it now. This week I noticed something funny. The skin over it seems awfully thick and tight."

Two days later, Dr. Perry found a small, hard mass in the upper outer quarter of Melissa's left breast. The skin over it was indeed thickened and retracted, dimpled inwards. In the left armpit he found two hard lymph nodes.

In another medical office three thousand miles away, David Carpenter was also hearing ominous news. David, 60 years old, had been a bus driver for the Los Angeles Transit System for twenty years. He had always enjoyed good health. Moderate in his habits, thin, and a nonsmoker, David had annual physical examinations at his union's health center. A routine proctoscopy test for rectal cancer was part of the exam, but he found the procedure unpleasant and uncomfortable. After the first time, he refused the proctoscopy.

"I never have any trouble there," he said. Carpenter still had no bowel symptoms, no constipation, no diarrhea, and no blood in his stool. But at this annual exam he reported that he had lost ten pounds in a few months without explanation. On examination his doctor found his liver to be enlarged, firm, and irregular. This time Carpenter agreed to the proctoscope exam. After positioning the patient, his doctor passed a narrow tube into the rectum and found a one-half-inch tumor growing from the rectal wall.

William Wilson, black, aged 45, was a farm worker outside Atlanta, Georgia. Wilson had started smoking when he was fourteen years old. For more than thirty years he had smoked two packages of cigarettes each day. He always had a morning cough, which he regarded as normal. This morning, however, something was different, his morning sputum tinged with bright red blood. The sight of blood frightened him, and he went that same morning to the General Hospital, where a chest X-ray was taken. The doctor called David into one of the cubicles off the main waiting room to give him the report. It wasn't good—there was a large spot on his left lung.

Melissa Miller, David Carpenter, and William Wilson had two things in common. The first was that they all had cancer. The second was that they had made serious errors in their own health care, errors that would shorten their lives and impair the quality of the life remaining to them.

Melissa Miller had ignored an important warning sign. She had felt something in her breast and had waited four long months, hoping it would go away by itself. During that time, spread to the regional lymph nodes in the armpit had occurred and the tumor had enlarged at its primary site in the breast. Not yet known, as she sat in her doctor's office, was that the malignant cells had spread to lymph nodes in the chest and to the pleura, the membrane around the lungs. Had she seen her doctor four months earlier, physical examination, X-ray of the breast (mammography), and biopsy could have elicited the diagnosis. With simple mastectomy at that point and plastic reconstruction if desired, Melissa's outlook would have been excellent for cure or many years of survival.

The four-month delay meant more extensive surgery, radical mastectomy, and lymph node dissection, followed by radiation accompanied by possible skin injury, bone marrow depression, and nausea. With distant spread of malignant cells, chemotherapy (potent anticancer drugs with noxious side effects) would have to be used. The quality and duration of life would be abbreviated. Melissa Miller ignored a warning sign. It was a fatal mistake.

David Carpenter also made a fatal mistake. He ignored a well-established preventive medicine tool, the annual proctoscopy exam for people, especially men, over age 40. Like hypertension, rectal cancer is a silent killer. It is often a slow-growing tumor affording ample time for early detection before spreading. Symptoms such as constipation, diarrhea, or blood in the stool may not occur until late in the course of the disease. The proctoscope, a ten-inch cylinder not much bigger in diameter than a human finger, is an instrument of great value. The examination takes one minute. More colon cancers occur within reach of the instrument than in any other comparable length of bowel. Simple office removal of an early malignancy gives close to 100 percent cure.

David Carpenter, however, faces a different outlook. Neglected rectal cancers may require abdominal surgery and permanent colostomy. Liver chemistries and biopsy of the liver proved that the cancer had spread to his liver, common with gastrointestinal cancer. As in Mrs. Miller's case, chemotherapy was necessary, and prospects dim.

William Wilson's fatal mistake was different. He did not ignore a symptom as did Melissa Miller, nor fail to have a routine preventive medical exam, as did David Carpenter. William's error lay in his continuing exposure to a potent carcinogen, inhaled cigarette smoke. We have known for two decades that cigarette smoking causes cancer of the lung. The five-year survival rate from the time the diagnosis of lung cancer is made is about 10 percent, no matter what form of therapy is used: thoracic surgery, radiation, or chemotherapy. In effect, treatment is almost without effect. The only solution is prevention—not smoking. Even smokers of many years' duration can decrease their risk of lung cancer to virtually that of nonsmokers, if they stop.

Cancer has not only a present but a past, a history we will look at in the next chapter.

NINE

THE HISTORY
OF CANCER

Cancer is not just a product of the twentieth century, although, as we shall see, the environment we have created to live in, our lifestyle and habits, our occupations, and the foods we do or don't eat, have activated a genetic trigger to fire more like a machine gun than a six-shooter.

The recorded history of the ancient Egyptians and Greeks speaks of cancer and primitive efforts to treat tumors. A reading of the fossil records of the earth's crust gives silent testimony to the existence of cancer in the dinosaur. Man has not been singled out. Cancer is widespread throughout all orders and phyla of animal life today.

In the modern era perhaps the most often quoted early observation was the story of the London chimney sweeps of the 18th century. Their incidence of scrotal cancer, an otherwise rare malady, was staggeringly high. In 1775 Dr. Percival Pott made the brilliant deduction that the high incidence resulted from the soot that sifted down inside the clothes of the sweeps and remained in prolonged contact with the scrotum.

In the nineteenth and twentieth centuries occupational patterns of cancer emerged in coal miners and chemical plant, asbestos, and radiation workers. One of the classic stories about radiation illustrates the insidious and varied nature of provoked cancers. In the early days of X-ray therapy, children who received thymus gland radiation came down with thyroid cancer decades later—about the same time as their radiologists were succumbing to leukemia. And the radiation in Hiroshima and Nagasaki created a kaleidoscope of tumors.

In retrospect it may seem naive to us but when radioactivity was a novelty, factory workers used radium paint to make wristwatch hands glow in the dark. To shape the points of their delicate brushes they habitually wet the brush tips with their tongues, transferring a microscopic dose of radioactive material to their mouths. It was decades later before an epidemic of mouth, lip, and tongue cancer erupted and led backward in time to the nearly forgotten production line practice that had started a lethal stopwatch ticking. What seemingly innocent daily exposure do we have, unknown to us, that will seem appallingly obvious in the year 2,000?

Geography as well as history offers other provocative clues. Why is it that Japanese residing in Hawaii or the West Coast of the United States are afflicted with stomach cancer at the same low incidence as Americans, while the disease remains epidemic in Japan? Jewish women from western Europe and North Africa differ greatly in their susceptibility to breast cancer. Once settled in Israel, their risk becomes equal to other Israelis.

In the past, a confusion of factors associated with cancer defied any logical pattern, serving only to confuse rather than clarify:

- Tobacco and lung cancer.
- Nitrosamines derived from foods such as bacon, bologna, etc., and stomach cancer.
- Genital herpes virus and cancer of the cervix.
- Diseases causing chronic tissue irritation: ulcerative colitis and large bowel cancer.
- Cirrhosis of the liver and liver cancer.
- Sex hormone differences: breast cancer rate much greater in women.
- Increasing age.
- Ethnic background: liver cancer in Chinese, esophageal cancer in Finns.
- Environmental hazards, including occupation.
- Genetic: "cancer families."

Although many squares remain to be filled in, with the emergence of the DNA oriented concept of cancer genesis a pattern has become clear. Genetic prevention and treatment of cancer may come in the

43

future. The time for cancer prevention by means of diet and environmental control is now.

Forty years after Berenblum's ground-breaking work on the initiation, latency, and promotion of cancer, the work of erecting a shield against cancer at last seems to be going forward, deep within the nuclei of our cells where the DNA spirals and ladders intertwine. Genetic research in the laboratories of Crick and Watson three decades ago led the way. Then in 1981 it fell to two epidemiologists, Richard Doll and Richard Peto, to organize that crazy quilt of observations about work, food, habits, and lifestyle into a meaningful fabric. They tell us that an astounding 80 percent of cancers are preventable.

We now have the knowledge of the biological mechanism and the social mechanics of cancer. Although much work remains, we now at least know where to begin.

TEN

CANCER SYMPTOMS

In the bad old days before we began to understand the genesis of cancer, the approach had to be something like a finger in the dike if a cancer was found early. If cancer was diagnosed late, the situation was more like closing the barn door after the cow was gone. It was that bad. Most people just waited for the axe to fall, hoping that it never would.

Lacking knowledge of prevention, doctors and the American Cancer Society had to focus their efforts on early detection, which offered the best chance of cure or at least longterm survival or palliation.

The effort was four-pronged. The first two involved publicizing the early symptoms of the common cancers and the need for prompt medical advice on the one hand, and on the other, campaigning for routine periodic cancer-oriented examinations in symptomfree individuals. Although it is difficult to quantify the effect of such campaigns, it is my feeling that they did achieve substantial success. The advice was good then, remains so today, and is worth repeating.

The seven warning signals emphasized by the American Cancer Society:

1. A change in bowel or bladder habits.
2. Any sore on the skin that does not heal.
3. Unexplained bleeding or discharge.

4. A lump in the breast or other part of the body.
5. Chronic indigestion or difficulty swallowing.
6. A change in a skin mole.
7. Chronic cough or hoarseness.

The advice of the American Cancer Society and of physicians in general has varied somewhat from time to time as our understanding of cancer, its varying timetable, and mechanisms of spread became more clear. Cancer-related check-ups must be individualized depending on age, sex, and individual risk factors. Cancer-related check-ups focus on the organs most likely, in a statistical sense, to develop tumors. In women the most common cancer is breast cancer, with lung, cervix, uterus and ovaries, and rectal cancer also important. In men, lung cancer is number one, with prostate and rectal cancer also prevalent. Other parts of the body, where cancer is less common, also merit attention: for example, the mouth, larynx and thyroid, lymph nodes and bone marrow, gastrointestinal and urinary tract, testicles, central nervous system, and skin.

For people without symptoms the American Cancer Society recommends a cancer-related check-up every three years between ages 20 and 40, and annually for ages 40 and over. People at higher risk than average for certain cancers may need more frequent examination; individuals with symptoms require prompt evaluation. The medical history should include a review of the individual's particular risks as suggested by his or her personal history of exposure, and advice on changes in habits and lifestyle. Personally I would set the dividing line at age 35, with a cancer-related check-up every one to two years prior to age 35 and annually thereafter. I would include cardiovascular risk factor analysis: blood pressure, cholesterol, blood sugar, and cigarette smoking.

Crucial in addition to the actual history and physical examination is the dialogue between doctor and patient, the discussion of family and personal history, social habits, the establishment of a good relationship between doctor and patient, the opportunity for patient education, and the repetition and reinforcement year after year of heart disease and cancer prevention information.

For women breast and pelvic exam (cervix, uterus, ovaries, Pap smear) and instruction in monthly self-examination of the breasts is vital.

46

Routine mammography is a controversial issue. The radiation itself increases the risk of breast cancer, especially in women under 35. The issue is in dispute for women between 40 and 50. Some authorities favor annual mammography in women over age 50. The matter is far from settled.

Recommended if you're over 35, essential if over 50: For males, prostate examination annually; for both sexes, proctoscopy for rectal cancer every one to two years. In the case of breast, pelvic, prostate, and rectal cancer, early detection improves the prospects of cure and decreases the dimensions of surgery if needed.

A chest X-ray detecting an asymptomatic early lung cancer does not improve survival. But the amount of radiation received from a chest plate is small and although not everyone agrees, a film at intervals of a few years may prove quite useful for comparison when uncertain findings appear on a current film. For showing trends in the size and shape of the heart and great arteries, periodic chest X-rays are an asset. Annual testing of a stool specimen for blood is simple, inexpensive, and valuable.

Public health organizations concerned about cost, practicality, and screening large numbers of people may recommend exams at longer intervals than one physician may to an individual for whom more frequent examination may be valuable.

The third effort by the medical community was research into the cause and prevention of cancer. One direction it took was the search for a *biologic marker*, a simple test that would be reliable, specific, sensitive, easy to do, inexpensive, reproducible from lab to lab and patient to patient, always positive for any malignancy, and negative in all other conditions. The search extended from microscopic analysis of handwriting to numerical calculations based on moment of birth. Scientific labs focused on blood analysis: some biochemical change, a protein fragment that should not be there, an aberration of amino acid structure—anything. Cancers are rapidly growing and metabolizing cell masses living off the body economy, commandeering blood vessels to supply them with oxygen, glucose, and amino acids; surely they must liberate some malignant metabolic waste products back into the blood, perhaps a change detectable in the blood occurring even before a clinical cancer develops or becomes evident. How exciting and important a finding that would be! In fact, an enormous number of substances were tested for and sought. Periodically premature reports would excite and then disappoint. We have yet to find a single biochemical or organic cancer marker.

The research was not without some worthwhile dividends. Some limited success was achieved:

CEA (carcinoembryonic antigen) is a glycoprotein that is increased in many patients having colon and rectum cancer. But not all patients with cancer of the colon have increased CEA, and some persons with other conditions do have it.

Alpha-fetoprotein, normal in the healthy fetus, is increased in most patients having cancer of the liver but, like CEA, it has insufficient specificity.

There are other markers having limited usefulness in specific tumors, but no single key to unlock cancer diagnosis has been found.

The fourth part of traditional cancer science was treatment—surgery, radiation, or chemotherapy—either alone or in combination. Some cures were achieved, but the physical and psychological mutilation could be as destructive as the disease itself, or even more so. The motives were honest and sincere but the available tools had limitations: the hazards of surgery, radiation injury to bone marrow and skin, or chemotherapy damage to marrow and liver function. Some excellent results were achieved, and all three treatments continue valid. Often, however, treatment produced little improvement, sometimes accelerating the downhill course.

All these avenues of diagnosis, research, and therapy must go on. An exciting, emerging technique, for example, is the use of monoclonal antibodies to target cancer cells for destruction while sparing normal cells. With this in mind, we are ready to look next at how big the cancer problem really is.

ELEVEN

CANCER
STATISTICS

Cancer. The word terrifies most of us. Although it is one disease, it is provoked by scores of agents and takes one hundred different forms, depending on the part of the body involved, age and sex, geography, ethnic and genetic factors, environment, occupation, habits, and diet.

For a long time a heated debate took place among scientists studying cancer: Was cancer one disease with a variety of forms? If so, laboratory research should be focused on finding the common denominator, the whole picture. Or were doctors seeing different diseases, clinical lookalikes with unrelated origins? Then study of each piece of the puzzle in people would make sense. Both sides of the argument were right.

While researchers were unraveling DNA in the lab, cancer patterns were under study by epidemiologists around the world. From this knowledge, each reader can learn his or her own risk and own role in prevention.

Let us look now at the cancer statistics for 1982. The American Cancer Society estimates that in 1982 death from cancer occurred in men as follows:

1. 34%—lung cancer.
2. 12%—colon and rectum cancer.
3. 10%—prostate cancer.

For females, the leading lethal cancers are:

1. 19%—breast cancer.
2. 16%—lung cancer.
3. 15%—colon and rectum cancer.
4. 11%—ovary, uterus, and cervix cancer.

In 1978, there were 1,927,788 deaths from all causes in the United States, with a death rate of 809.9 per 100,000 population. Of this number, cardiovascular diseases were number one with 49.2 percent of all deaths. Cancer was second, with 20.6 percent of all deaths, a death rate of 169.9 per 100,000 population, or a total of 396,992 deaths from cancer.

For each person the chance of cancer depends on many variables—to begin with, sex, age, and type of cancer.

Males of All Ages (1978)

Cancer	Deaths
Lung	71,006
Colon and Rectum	25,696
Prostate	21,674
Pancreas	11,010
Stomach	8,529

No. 1 Lethal Cancer—Males

Age	Cancer	No. of Deaths
0–34	Leukemia	1,377
35–54	Lung	10,124
55–74	Lung	46,049
75 and above	Lung	14,646

No. 2 and No. 3 Lethal Cancers—Males

Age	No.	Cancer	No. of Deaths
0–34		Male cancer deaths are relatively rare, with up to a few hundred occurring from brain and central nervous system, bone, kidney, Hodgkin's disease, testicle, and melanoma (skin) cancers.	

Age	No.	Cancer	No. of Deaths
35–54	2	Colon and Rectum	2,462
	3	Pancreas	1,262
55–74	2	Colon and Rectum	13,717
	3	Prostate	9,047
75 and above	2	Prostate	12,298
	3	Colon and Rectum	9,325

In the age group 35 and over, stomach cancer, bladder cancer, brain and central nervous system cancer, and leukemia are the fourth or fifth most common.

Just from these initial data it is apparent that different cancers have specific patterns of occurrence with respect to age, information that should be useful in guiding cancer research.

There are comparable data for female deaths from the five leading cancers of women by age group for 1978.

Females of All Ages (1978)

Cancer	Deaths
Breast	34,329
Colon and Rectum	27,573
Lung	24,080
Uterus	10,842
Ovary	10,651

No. 1 Lethal Cancer—Females

Age	Cancer	No. of Deaths
0–15	Leukemia	411
15–34	Breast	585
35–54	Breast	8,205
55–74	Breast	17,403
75 and above	Colon and Rectum	12,626

Age	No.	Cancer	No. of Deaths
0–34		Similar to male	
35–54	2	Lung	4,679
	3	Colon and Rectum	2,210
55–74	2	Lung	14,463
	3	Colon and Rectum	12,551
75 and above	2	Breast	8,129
	3	Lung	4,819

Cancers of the uterus and ovary occupy fourth and fifth place between ages 35 and 74.

In 1978 there were 215,997 cancer deaths in males and 180,995 in females. Both were second only to cardiovascular diseases. For males of all ages cancer is consistently the second most common cause of death, with the exception of males aged 15 to 34, in whom accidents, homicide, and suicide precede cancer. For females, cancer is also consistently the second most common cause of death, with the exception of females aged 35 to 54, in whom cancer is the number-one cause and females 75 and above, in whom cancer is the number-three cause.

Cancer Deaths

Males	
Age	No. of Deaths
35–54	26,942
55–74	120,955
75 and above	62,863

Females	
Age	No. of Deaths
35–54	27,896
55–74	90,016
75 and above	58,656

Cancer rates charted for specific organs in females and males between 1930 and 1978 show some very interesting trends. In females the cancer rates for uterus, stomach, and liver have shown a gradual downward trend. For breast, colon and rectum, ovary, pancreas, and stomach, there has been very little change. The dramatic change has occurred in the rate of lung cancer. Between 1930 and 1965 there was very little change, the rate of female lung cancer deaths varying between 3 and 6 per 100,000. From 1965 to 1978, the incidence of lethal lung cancer in women rose sharply and dramatically, with 19 to 20 cases per 100,000 in 1978. With the rate of breast cancer stable for 50 years at about 25 to 27 deaths per 100,000 per year, the curve for lung cancer will soon cross and surpass that for breast cancer, taking over the number-one spot sometime between 1983 and 1985.

For males the curves for most cancer deaths have been fairly stable for the last 50 years, showing only minor increase or no change at all for cancer of the esophagus, bladder, pancreas, leukemia, liver, prostate, colon, and rectum. The two exceptions are stomach cancer, the incidence of which dropped from 37 cases per 100,000 in 1930 in a steady decline to 9 cases per 100,000 in 1978, and lung cancer, which rose in a straight line from 5 or 6 cases per 100,000 in 1930 to 71 cases per 100,000 in 1978. The reasons for the drop in stomach cancer are not entirely clear, although they may be related to changes in food processing and preservation during that period. The increase in lung cancer, as we all know, is a result of cigarette smoking.

In 1982, a total of 835,000 new cases of cancer and 430,000 deaths from cancer were expected in the United States. New cases and deaths for specific organs should break down as follows:

Organ	New Cases	Deaths
Colon and Rectum	123,000	57,100
Lung	129,000	111,000
Breast	112,900	37,300
Cervix	16,000	7,100
Uterus	39,000	3,000
Ovary	18,000	11,400
Prostate	73,000	23,300

In general, the number of new cancer cases is about double the number of cancer deaths. For specific organs the ratio varies. For breast cancer, the death to new case rate is about 33 percent, while for lung cancer it is about 86 percent. Such relationships tell us that tumors vary in virulence, ease of early diagnosis, and effectiveness of treatment.

It is interesting to look at cancer death rates per 100,000 population for different countries. Data were collected from 42 countries in 1976 and 1977. Of the 42 countries, the United States ranked seventeenth highest for males and nineteenth highest for females, with 213.6 male and 136.3 female deaths per 100,000 population. With the exception of Uruguay, which was number one (male and female) with 294.6 male and 180.3 female deaths per 100,000 the top ten were all in western Europe. Whether differences in diagnosing and reporting play a role in the statistics is difficult to say. It is interesting to speculate on the high cancer rates in Uruguay. The diet, high in beef, could be at fault, yet Argentina on the same diet ranked nineteenth (male) and eighteenth (female). Honduras, Nicaragua, Thailand, and the Philippines occupied the lowest positions for both male and female. Again it is interesting to speculate whether characteristics of the diet, the general economic status of the countries, and the absence of industrialization played significant roles.

The lowest incidence of cancer deaths for males was in Honduras with 24.5 per 100,000, and for females in Thailand with 24.8 per 100,000.

Looking now only at United States cancer deaths, for colon and rectum the United States ranked male: sixteenth with 26.2 per 100,000 and female: fifteenth with 20.2 per 100,000. For lung cancer, the United States ranked male: sixth with 68.1 per 100,000, and female: fifth with 17.2 per 100,000. For breast cancer, the United States ranked fourteenth with 27.3 per 100,000; for cancer of the uterus thirtieth with 8.9 per 100,000; and for prostate cancer, twelfth with 22.3 per 100,000.

The five-year cancer survival rates for white males and females between 1964 and 1973 is also of interest in telling us about the differences between different tumors:

Five-Year Survival (in percent)

Organ	Percent Overall	If Localized At Time Of Diagnosis	If Spread At Time Of Diagnosis
Colon and Rectum	47	77	29
Breast	68	88	50
Cervix	59	82	41
Uterus	79	90	40
Ovary	35	81	20
Prostate	63	77	39

It is also interesting to look at tumors of various organs in terms of whether they were local or showed regional or distant spread at the time of diagnosis. For cases between 1970 and 1973:

At Time of Diagnosis (in percent)

Organ	Local	Regional	Distant
Colon and Rectum	44	26	25
Lung	17	22	48
Breast	48	41	9
Uterus	63	23	12
Ovary	25	6	64
Prostate	61	13	21

The figures show that some tumors make their presence known early, before regional or distant spread. For other tumors the first symptom may reflect distant spread, which accounts for lower survival rates. That is particularly true, for example, in the cases of cancer of the lung and ovary.

Improvements in survival presumably reflect earlier diagnosis or better treatment. Compare the five-year survival in white patients from 1960 to 1963 with that from 1970 to 1973. For prostate cancer the survival improved from 50 to 63 percent at the five-year mark. For cancer of the uterus the survival rate went from 73 to 81 percent, for the cervix from 58 to 64 percent, for the colon and rectum from 41 to 48 percent, for the breast from 63 to 68 percent, for the ovary from 32 to 36 percent, for the lung from 8 to 10 percent.

For 1982, the 835,000 new cases of cancer include 413,000 in males and 422,000 in females. The 430,000 deaths from cancer include 233,000 in males and 197,000 in females.

Age-adjusted cancer death rates per 100,000 population for the white population show that in 1950 the rate was 125.4 for males and 130.9 for females, and rose steadily for males, reaching a high of 160.0 in 1977, with the greatest rise coming between 1955 and 1960 and smaller rises between 1960 and 1965 and 1965 to 1970. For females the 1950 rate of 130.9 rose to 137.4 in 1955 and then dropped to 109.5 in 1960. It has remained stable at approximately that rate since then, until 1977, when the rate was 108.3. For black men and women, parallel changes have occurred, but at higher levels since 1960. The 1950 rate for nonwhite males was 125.8, which rose to 205.4 by 1977.

For nonwhite females, the 1950 rate of 131.0 decreased to 122.4 by 1977.

The overall age-adjusted cancer death rates per 100,000 population for all organs, sexes, and races in the United States between 1950 and 1977 shows a rate of 125.4 in 1950, which remained almost unchanged until 1965, when it was 127.0, and has shown a gradual, small increase since then, reaching 133.0 in 1977.

An important factor to recall in looking at these data is that some refer to the number of new cases and some to deaths. Data are also organized in terms of different organ systems, different ages, and different sexes, and comparisons are made among different countries and different periods of time. Different factors may affect these data, such as the completeness of data collection, the accuracy of death certificate diagnoses from which much of the data are obtained, differing diagnostic abilities of medical attendants, the difference in cancer incidence between the sexes and between different ethnic and racial groups, differences in screening methods and methods of treatment, and more widespread use of medical care by different populations. Increasing life expectancy may make certain diagnoses appear to increase although that can be statistically corrected.

Trends that remain after keeping such factors in mind suggest possible cancer causes. For example, the decrease in stomach cancer during the last 35 years may be due to preserving food by refrigeration rather than by pickling and salting. Decreases in cervical cancer during the same period may be due to use of the Pap test. Detecting and treating precancerous changes decreases the number of new cases and the death rate from cervical cancer. For breast cancer, regular examination will decrease the death rate.

Because the National Center for Health Statistics, the American Cancer Society, and the National Cancer Institute use somewhat different statistical methods for gathering and analyzing data, exact numbers and percentages may vary slightly from study to study. In addition some agencies do and others do not use statistical corrections to correct for the changing numbers of people of a given age. Nevertheless, the findings are comparable.

The changes in lung cancer incidence are attributed to cigarette smoking. Changes in colon and rectal cancer rates may be affected by improved diagnosis, causing an apparent increase in incidence. That in turn may lead to a lower death rate because of early diagnosis and improved methods of treatment. Also, issues of changing dietary practices of the population may influence the rates of colon and rectal cancer.

For prostate cancer, longer male life expectancy and increased discovery results in an increased number of cases. Cancer of the uterus (excluding the cervix) increased during the first half of the 1970s, which may correlate with the increased use of estrogen at that time to treat menopausal symptoms.

About 25 percent of all Americans will develop cancer at some time during their lives. About 20 percent of all Americans will die of cancer, the other 5 percent with cancer from noncancerous causes. During the last 35 years the incidence of cancer has decreased among women under 45 years of age. It has increased among men over 45.

Again, keeping in mind that the exact numbers, percentages, and rates may vary slightly and that such variations do not profoundly affect the use of the data, the next step involves some thoughtful, even bold, deductions; theories to test; and directions for research. Integrating information about human behavior with all the tables and numbers, trend lines on graphs, and percentages can tell us much about what causes cancer. We have not changed genetically in the last 50 years, yet some cancers have diminished and others have swelled to frightening proportions. Some of the factors affecting the statistics have been hinted at. In Parts III and IV of this book we will systematically examine our lifestyles, habits, environment, the foods we eat, the air we breathe—in fact, the chemistry of life around and within us, especially as it has changed over the last half century. From matching changes in human behavior to the shifting patterns of cancer and by sorting to find parallels and pairs and causes and effects, clues may surface about how to adapt our lives.

THE CANCER-
PREVENTION
DIET

TWELVE

BETA-CAROTENE

The Beta Unit

What is a *beta unit*? A beta unit is an accurate, if seemingly unscientific, measure of the cancer prevention potential in one average, ordinary portion of a food high in beta-carotene (provitamin A). The capability to prevent cancer may reside in beta-carotene itself or in some unknown substance in the same foods as beta-carotene.

Can we justify using something as vague and variable as an average ordinary portion of food? In this case, yes, providing we keep our goal solidly in mind.

First, because we are not certain of the exact nature of the mysterious anticancer substance, we cannot use the ordinary scientific measurements of milligrams, grams or cubic centimeters.

Second, we must heed the distinction between precision and accuracy. It is quite possible to be very precise at the same time that one is totally inaccurate. For example, if we say that the distance from the earth to the sun is 99.54321 million miles, we are giving a very precise figure that is totally inaccurate. If, on the other hand, we say that distance is 93 million miles, our accuracy is excellent, although the precision is acceptably unprecise. Because we are interested in getting on with our cancer prevention diet as soon as possible, what we are after is accuracy. That is not to say that we are uninterested in further defining the anticancer substance. There are studies in progress to reveal its identity, nature, and mechanism of action, down to the molecular structure. Exploration of its properties may open doorways to further cancer prevention and treatment.

Third, much information has been derived from the laboratory dish and the experimental animal. But for our purposes the best data have been collected from epidemiology, the medical science devoted to the study of great masses of people, their diet, habits, health, and disease. It is epidemiology that supplied us with the clue about the relationship between diet and cancer. It is to epidemiology that we must look for the guidelines to apply that knowledge.

A portion of food will, of course, vary from day to day on the family table, or from restaurant to restaurant. The size of a portion will depend very much on the age, sex, physical activity, ethnic origin, and the country where the eater lives. But practically speaking there are limits to how small or large that portion may be. Most of the epidemiologic data showing a beneficial relationship between eating beta-carotene foods and lower cancer rates did not define the amount of food eaten. A study begun today asking large numbers of people to measure and eat precise quantities of foods over a period of several years would have very few takers and almost no hope of successful conclusion. Fortunately we are dealing with a cancer protective effect that occurs in diets spontaneously chosen by some people, because of either availability of the foods or personal taste preferences, but not ingested in quantities that are unusually high by any reasonable standard. Consciously consuming excessive quantities of foods beyond the normal satisfaction of hunger would probably be in vain. It is likely that beyond a certain level there is a maximum ability of the body to absorb, transport, and utilize such substances.

The CBA
(Cancer-Blocking Agent)

If the cancer-blocking agent is a vitamin or enzyme, the body requires only minute quantities of such substances, which act by promoting other biochemical reactions within the body.

People who consume little of the cancer-blocking agent will be at the greatest risk for the development of cancer. There is probably a middle ground of people who consume moderate quantities of CBAs and develop cancer at an intermediate rate. The maximum CBA potential occurs in individuals who regularly consume CBA foods on a daily or almost daily basis. The data available do not suggest that beyond a certain point additional quantities of CBA foods produce greater benefit. Most biological phenomena have optimum zones of function beyond which there is no further benefit, but even potential toxicity.

In short, the data we have suggest that ordinary people regularly consuming reasonable portions of CBA foods benefit from significantly lower cancer rates. The effect appears to be universal in every part of the globe, in every ethnic group, at every socioeconomic level for which observations of diet and cancer rates have been made. The method of preparation of food does not appear to affect its CBA content. Whether consumed raw or eaten cooked, it appears not to matter, although prolonged cooking at very high temperatures should probably be avoided because extremes of heat do affect some substances with biological activity.

The beta unit is one ordinary portion of one of the CBA foods.

The Cancer Prevention and Weight Management Diet

We will discuss food groups, grams, and calories, fat, protein, carbohydrate, vitamins and minerals, and food lists so you can measure the beta-carotene diet system against some diet guidelines with which we are already familiar. But there will be no calorie counting, no gram calculating, no bizarre diet distortions, no diet that is unpalatable and unlivable for the long term, no diet that is inconsistent with the best health information that we now have as it applies to heart trouble, high blood pressure, or diabetes, no lengthy diet lists or rigid, restrictive menus. Read this section and then forget the details, the numbers, the counting, the calculating and computing, taking away with you only the concept. Indeed, after a few days of occasionally referring to this part of the book, the First and Second Rules of Tens and Twelves (see Chapter 14) will become so much second nature that your daily food selection will become an automatic, healthful habit. Flexible alternatives allow you to choose according to your own tastes and preferences within a dietary system that will give you the benefit of our most up-to-date data on cancer prevention, preservation of cardiovascular health, and achievement of the best body weight for you.

Food lists are not meant to be exhaustive of every variant fruit and vegetable on the planet but will be representative of most of the foods we are accustomed to eat. Substitution of foods not on the list is not only permitted but encouraged if they please your palate more. Only your common sense and common knowledge will be needed to identify the group to which the food belongs.

Diets can be looked at from the point of view of their calorie content, their protein, carbohydrate and fat content, and their vitamin and mineral content. Fats can be broken down into saturated and unsaturated fat; and then there are cholesterol and fiber content. But calories or grams are not visible to the naked eye. Very few of us have the inclination to dissect our foods in such a manner, and that is a major failing of most diets. We eat foods, not mathematical symbols, so we will be dealing with the common English names of foods and their common classification into vegetables, fruits, grains, milk, and meat products. The calorie and gram information you will read is for background information only. They need not be remembered, however, for they are built into the bottom line of food portion choices.

Grams

A word in passing about grams and kilograms, two measures of weight with which most of us in the United States are not entirely comfortable. The language of science is expressed in these units, and in a moment we can familiarize ourselves with them. One gram is a rather small unit of weight. It takes 454 grams to equal one pound; a rough approximation is 500 grams to the pound. A kilogram is 1,000 grams and works out to approximately 2.2 pounds. An average-size man of 154 pounds, in the metric system weighs 70 kilograms. A gram, however, is mammoth compared to some of the weights of substances that have potent biologic effect. Most of the time in medical science we talk about milligrams, abbreviated *mg*. One milligram is one thousandth of a gram, that is, it takes 1,000 milligrams to equal one gram. Even smaller than the milligram is the microgram, which is abbreviated with the Greek letter mu (μ) followed by a small g. It takes 1,000 micrograms to equal one milligram.

Planning a diet must begin with knowledge of our protein, fat, carbohydrate, and calorie requirements.

Protein

A normal, healthy adult requires about 0.8 gram of protein per kilogram of body weight per day. For a 70-kilogram person, his average daily intake of protein should be about 70 × 0.8, or 56 grams of protein. In actual practice one can vary this substantially from day to day but there is no real benefit in taking large amounts of protein regularly nor is there any real problem with sometimes taking smaller amounts of protein. Marked protein deprivation over a period of weeks to months does have an adverse effect on the body, which will lack the building blocks (amino acids) provided by dietary protein for the repair and maintenance of the body's own protein structure and needs. A slender woman of 110 pounds, or 50 kilograms, will need somewhat less protein—in this case 40 grams, while a tall, muscular man of 198 pounds, or 90 kilograms, will need 72 grams of protein. The average woman or man of average body build needs approximately 50 to 60 grams of protein per day.

Larger amounts of protein are simply converted by the body to sugar or fat. Even huge amounts of protein can be handled by the normal liver and kidney but the metabolic truth is that a little is good, but more is *not* better. Aside from increasing blood sugar and the size of fat depots and contributing to overweight, excessive protein is damaging in people with liver and kidney disorders and gout. Diets high in animal protein are high in animal fat, the high-risk food for heart disease and cancer.

Calories

Before looking at fat and carbohydrate requirements, we must deal with calories. A calorie is simply a measure of the energy available, the biologic energy content of the various types of foodstuffs. Looking at charts of calorie requirements tends to be unnecessarily confusing because they are set up with so many variables depending on age, sex, energy expenditure, work, pregnancy, and breast feeding. A simple rule of thumb will cover the basic calorie needs of healthy adult men and women. Healthy adult males require approximately 2,500 calories per day, which may vary by a few hundred calories per day depending on height, weight, age, and level of physical activity. For women the key figure is 2,000 calories per day, again varying with age, height, weight, level of physical activity, pregnancy, or lactation. The modest differences in caloric need from individual to individual are accommodated, as you will see when we come to the details of the *portion-oriented diet*. We will also take into account whether an individual is at or above desired body weight.

Carbohydrate and protein both contain 4 calories per gram. A level teaspoon of sugar contains 4½ grams of carbohydrate, or 18 calories. Fat is much higher in its caloric content, more than double that of protein and carbohydrate. Each gram of fat has 9 calories.

Now that we have established the protein and caloric need of a healthy person, we can figure the fat and carbohydrate needs.

Fat

Most Americans in the past consumed about 40 percent of their total calories in the form of fat, and too high a proportion of that in the form of saturated, or animal, fat. Given the strong evidence relating animal fat to heart disease and new evidence relating dietary fat to cancer, health authorities are now recommending a reduction in fat consumption from 40 to 30 percent of total calories. That is a conservative drop, well within the capabilities of most of us, given our new understanding of its importance. A percentage as low as 20 may be forthcoming, with the bottom line on fat consumption depending on the difficulty of breaking traditional diet habits, the palatability of foods, and the need for some fat in the diet. Taste preference may be a result of childhood conditioning; extremely low-fat diets are unpalatable to many people. Many flavorings and spices are fat, not water, soluble, so aroma and flavor require some fat as a vehicle. In addition, lower percentages are difficult because of the frequent association in foods of fat with needed fat soluble vitamins (A and D), calcium, and protein (although virtually fat-free vegetarian diets can be constructed to provide the necessary protein building blocks).

Fats can be broken down into three types: saturated fats derived from animal sources, and monounsaturated and polyunsaturated fats derived from vegetable, fruit, and seed sources. For example, olives are high in monounsaturated fat and sunflower seeds in polyunsaturated fat. The main culprit in the genesis of cardiovascular disease and cancer is saturated fat of animal origin, but unsaturated fat in excess is a cause of cancer, too. Fats from animal sources should be limited to no more than 10 percent of total calories in the diet.

66

For our 2,500 calorie per day man, 30 percent maximum for total fat means no more than 750 calories of fat and, of this, only 250 calories from animal-fat sources. For our 2,000 calorie per day woman, 30 percent gives a figure of 600 calories per day for total fat and, of this, 200 calories per day for animal fat.

Cholesterol
Cholesterol intake should be limited to under 300 milligrams per day, the cholesterol content of a single egg yolk. Other foods high in cholesterol include red meats, dairy products, such as butter, cheese, or ice cream, and shellfish, including shrimp, clams, and lobster.

Grams/Calories and Fat/Protein/Carbohydrate
We can now calculate the total grams and calories of fat, protein, and carbohydrate for our Standard Adult Male (SAM) and Standard Adult Lady (SAL), shown in Tables I and II.

TABLE I:

SAM

	Grams	Calories
Fat	83.33	750
Protein	56.0	224
Carbohydrate	381.5	1,526
	Total	2,500

This amount of carbohydrate is well in excess of the minimum (60 grams per day) required to prevent ketosis, an abnormal metabolic state due to tissue fat breakdown. Prolonged or profound ketosis can cause major damage.

TABLE II:

SAL

	Grams	Calories
Fat	66.66	600
Protein	50.0	200
Carbohydrate	300.0	1,200
	Total	2,000

The figures presuppose that the individuals are normal, healthy adult men and women who are neither underweight nor overweight and who are using the number of calories consumed per day.

The proportions of fat, protein and carbohydrate certainly will vary in the diet from day to day and from individual to individual. Substantial variations, particularly for short periods, pose no threat to health whatsoever. Many individuals consume higher amounts of protein, lower amounts of carbohydrate, and greater or lesser amounts of fat. Growing children, pregnant or breast-feeding women, the very elderly, the bedridden, those doing heavy physical labor, and people with various disorders such as diabetes may vary substantially from these figures. They do, nevertheless, reflect food intake patterns common to normal, healthy adults.

Weight Loss
To lose one pound your caloric balance sheet must show a 3,500 calorie deficit, that is, your body must use up 3,500 more calories for its metabolic and energy needs than you are consuming. A simple rule of thumb is that a 500 calorie deficit per day will produce a one pound weight loss per week, or a thousand calorie deficit per day will produce a two pound weight loss per week. With SAM and SAL's normal energy requirements, to lose two pounds a week means decreasing SAM's daily calorie consumption from 2,500 to 1,500 calories, and SAL's from 2,000 to 1,000 calories. Their daily vitamin and mineral requirements are listed in Chapter 3.

A person on an absolute fast with zero calorie intake can lose a maximum of about 0.7 pounds per day. This may seem surprisingly little to you. The figure is simple to derive. SAM requires about 2,500 calories per day to sustain baseline metabolic functions and modest physical activity. A net deficit of 3,500 calories below baseline requirements is equivalent to a loss of one pound of true weight. The deficit produced by using 2,500 calories in a day during which no food is consumed is 0.71 pounds. SAL requires about 2,000 calories per day for metabolic maintenance and normal physical activity; the weight loss would be 0.57 pounds per day.

What is the explanation for the impressive weight loss seen on the very first day in many popular diets? Most of that loss is water (see Chapter 4). Individuals who are substantially overweight tend to retain water for a number of reasons. There is increased water content within the cells (the intracellular fluid) and in the microscopic spaces between the cells (the intercellular fluid). Additional water is held in loose chemical attachment to fat in fat depots. Excess water may be found within the circulatory system, especially because individuals eating a lot of food and fat often consume large amounts of salt, which requires fluid for dilution to a concentration acceptable to the body. The abrupt decrease in food, fat, water, and salt intake associated with most popular diets, and the ensuing tissue breakdown releases a gush of water, doubling or tripling urine volume.

The minimum amount of urine needed for the excretion of body wastes is 600 cc per day; 1,000 cc (one liter in metric measurement) equals about one quart, the volume measurement in daily American usage—600 cc, then, is a little over half a quart per day. Most people normally produce a less concentrated urine, about 1,000 to 1,500 cc per day. By responding to thirst we consume more water than essential, creating a more dilute urine and less work for the kidneys, the organ that concentrates the urine. One quart weighs approximately 2.2 pounds. An individual who increases his urine output from 1,000 to 2,500 cc per day by a dietary change freeing retained water will lose 2½ quarts of fluid, 5.5 pounds, in a single day. Additional water is lost with respiration, perspiration, and in the stool. A loss of 5.5 pounds in one day is impressive to anyone who ever struggled to lose one pound per week. Word rapidly spreads—a new miracle diet has been born. Disillusion comes weeks to months later as weight is regained. The (unphysiologic) state of dehydration provoked by the diet prompts increased fluid intake. The diet is terminated because of unpleasant and even dangerous metabolic derangements. Diets aimed at weight loss alone, ignoring what should be the primary objective—good health—cannot be sustained for very long. Previous eating habits supervene and the lost weight is regained, and frequently more.

Normal Weight
What constitutes normal weight has long been a subject of debate. The range of values for each height is so wide in some tables that it is impractical for an individual to judge where he stands. Attempts to simplify—small, medium, or large frame charts, weight at age 21, or thickness of abdominal skinfolds—only further confuse.

Table III is realistic. Measurements given are without shoes and in very light or no clothing. For males 5′2″ to 6′2″ the weight range is from 123 to 171 pounds, with a four pound increase for each inch of height. The range at each height is from 12 pounds below to 12 pounds above the average weight (the Third Rule of Twelves—see Chapter 14). Only conscientious appraisal of your frame type, presence of belly tissue folds, recollection of your weight at age 21, and honest self-appraisal can tell you where you belong within that range. If you are unable to determine it, you should shoot for the average weight noted.

For women between heights 5'0" and 6'0" the average weight (Table III) varies from 107 to 149 pounds with a three to four pound increase per inch of height and a range of 10 pounds below to 10 pounds above (the Third Rule of Tens).

TABLE III

Height	Weight in Pounds	
	Males (plus or minus 12 lbs.)	Females (plus or minus 10 lbs.)
5'0"		107
5'1"		110
5'2"	123	113
5'3"	127	116
5'4"	131	119
5'5"	135	122
5'6"	139	125
5'7"	143	129
5'8"	147	133
5'9"	151	137
5'10"	155	141
5'11"	159	145
6'0"	163	149
6'1"	167	
6'2"	171	

If you're good in math and like formulas, try the following to find your ideal weight. Multiply your height in inches by 2.54 to get your height in centimeters. Move the decimal point two places to the left to get your height in meters. Multiply your height in meters by

70

itself and multiply that answer by 22 to get your ideal weight in kilograms. Multiply by 2.2 to get the ideal weight in pounds.

Example:	5'10" tall	= 70" (male)
	70 × 2.54	= 177.8 cm.
	177.8 cm.	= 1.778 meters
	1.778 × 1.778	= 3.16 (approx.)
	3.16 × 22	= 69.52 Kg.
	69.52 × 2.2	= 153 pounds (approx.)
	Range: 153 ± 12	= 141 to 165 pounds

This is a scientific formula devised in 1972 for correlating height and weight. Women can use a multiplier of 20 or 21 instead of 22. However, the commonsense index about how you realistically look and feel should be applied in a sober moment to assess whether you are overweight.

Recapitulation

A true loss of one to two pounds per week can be achieved by reducing caloric intake 500 to 1,000 calories per day, with a diet providing 50 grams of protein for repair, maintenance and growth, at least 60 grams of carbohydrate for energy (no less because of the ketosis induced by fat breakdown in carbohydrate deprived diets) and small amounts of fat: 30 percent (some say 20 percent) of total calories with a 10–10–10 percent distribution among saturated, monounsaturated, and polyunsaturated fat.

THIRTEEN

DIETARY GUIDELINES

- Choose foods from a variety of food groups every day. Include fruits, vegetables (including legumes—peas and beans), nuts and seeds, whole grain products (breads and cereals), skim milk, poultry, fish, egg whites, and a minimum of lean red meats.
- Avoid overweight and significant underweight.
- Avoid too much fat, especially saturated fat (fat from animal sources), and cholesterol. Avoid fatty meats, egg yolks, organ meats such as liver or brain, cooking fats of animal origin, and coconut and palm oil. Use other cooking methods in preference to frying. (Infrequently, once or twice a week, deviations from this diet pattern are not considered harmful.)
- As a source of carbohydrate, complex carbohydrates, such as those found in whole grain products, fruits and vegetables, legumes, and nuts are preferable to simple sugars. Avoid sweet-tasting foods.
- Avoid excessive salt, pickled foods, smoked and cured foods, and alcohol.

Fat consumption should be no more than 30 percent of total caloric intake (10 percent saturated, 10 percent monounsaturated, 10 percent polyunsaturated). Carbohydrate should represent about 58 percent of energy intake (48 percent complex carbohydrates, and no more than 10 percent simple refined/processed sugars). Cholesterol consumption should be a maximum of 300 milligrams per day. Salt consumption should be much less than 5 grams per day.

Increase fruits, vegetables and whole grains. Use poultry, fish and lean meats only. Use low-fat or nonfat milk and milk products.

Decrease simple sugars and salt. Decrease foods high in total fat, particularly animal fat. Decrease consumption of butter, cheese, egg yolks and fatty meats.

The Food Groups

Group A—Vegetables

1. Beta-carotene vegetables
2. Legumes—peas and beans
3. Nuts and seeds
4. Other vegetables

Group B—Fruits

Group C—Grains (breads and cereals) and starchy vegetables

Group D—Milk and Meats

Group X—Other permitted foods

Group Y—Other foods that may be eaten infrequently

A few simple definitions of some common words are in order to be sure we are using them similarly. Although our definitions might not satisfy a botanist, they are what we understand the words to mean in everyday language.

A. Vegetables: edible plants, generally growing in or on the ground or on vines. We eat the leaves or roots, sometimes the seeds and pulp.
1. cruciferous vegetables—plants of the mustard family whose flowers have four parts forming a cross, including mustards, cabbages, cresses, broccoli, cauliflower, and brussels sprouts.
2. legumes—peas and beans; pods with seeds.
3. seeds—the part of a flowering plant from which a new plant can grow (sunflower) and nuts—the dried seeds of trees or bushes, encased in a tough shell or kernel (almonds, pecans).
4. leaves (spinach) and roots (carrots).

B. Fruits—grow on trees, shrubs, and bushes, vinelike; the seeds and surrounding pulp or flesh (apples and oranges).
C. Grains—the small, edible nuggets of cereal plants (wheat, rice and corn) and starchy vegetables (potatoes).
D. Milk (dairy products) and meats (from animals and fish).

With these working definitions in mind we will now list the specific foods in each group. Remember, the lists are not exhaustive, but represent the common foods consumed by most Americans. As a rule, foods not on the list, but obviously belonging to a particular group, can be substituted.

GROUP A1
Beta-Carotene Vegetables

Dark Green Leafy Vegetables	Dark Yellow Vegetables	Cruciferous Vegetables
spinach	carrots	cabbage cauliflower
		broccoli brussels sprouts

GROUP A2
Legumes

peas	kidney beans	tofu
pinto beans	lentils	green beans
lima beans	soy beans	chickpeas

GROUP A3
Nuts and Seeds

almonds	sunflower
walnuts	pumpkin
peanuts	safflower, etc.
pecans, etc.	

GROUP A4
Other Vegetables

asparagus	eggplants	peppers
beets	lettuce	radishes
celery	mushrooms	tomatoes
cucumbers	onions	turnips

GROUP B
Fruits and Juices

apples	blackberries	grapefruits	pears
apricots	canteloupe	grapes	pineapples
bananas	honeydew melons	lemons	plums
raspberries	cherries	oranges	prunes
blueberries	dates	tangerines	raisins
strawberries	figs	peaches	watermelons

GROUP C
Grains and Starchy Vegetables

bread	tortillas
rolls	pasta
crackers	noodles
biscuits	rice
muffins	corn
cereals (preferably whole grain)	potatoes
pizza	bulgur wheat

GROUP D
Milk, Meat, Poultry, and Fish

skim milk or lowfat milk	veal
soft margarine	poultry
lowfat cheese	fish
ice milk	egg whites

GROUP X
Other Permitted Foods

coffee (moderate quantities)	corn oil
tea	sunflower oil
lemon	safflower oil
spices	olive oil (moderate quantities)
vinegar	peanut butter (moderate quantities)

GROUP Y

Other Foods Permitted *RARELY*

sweet foods	creamy salad dressings	flavored yogurt (high in sugar)
soft drinks	pickled foods	
excessive salt	smoked foods	potato chips and similar snacks
bakery products	saccharin	
chocolate	jams and jellies	avocados
mayonnaise		

Foods High in Cholesterol and/or Saturated Fats

palm and coconut oil	red meat
lard or other animal fats for cooking	beef
gravy	lamb
egg yolks	pork
creamed products	ham
ice cream	bacon
cheese	luncheon meats, or cold cuts
soup	sausages
butter	hot dogs
tripe	hamburgers
shellfish	organ meats

Alcohol can be used minimally, tobacco not at all.

Monounsaturated fat is found in foods such as olives, and polyunsaturated fat in corn. Vegetable margarines that have been solidified by partial hydrogenation (which must be on the product ingredient label) are partially saturated fats. It appears that cholesterol and saturated fat are most important in the genesis of cardiovascular disease, but it is saturated fat that is most important as a cause of cancer. However, for individuals on low saturated fat diets, consumption of large amounts of monounsaturated and polyunsaturated fats may provoke cancer.

FOURTEEN

THE FIRST RULE OF TENS AND TWELVES

William Sidney Porter (O. Henry) achieved fame with his many short stories about the foibles of man and the ironies of life. Perhaps you remember *Two Thanksgiving Day Gentlemen,* the story of the elderly men who met at a park bench once a year at Thanksgiving. One year, the first man, once well-to-do, was down in the world and starving. Out of respect for their custom, with his last dollar he bought the second man, a drifter, his Thanksgiving dinner. The second man, this year already the overstuffed beneficiary of one free dinner complete from turkey to pumpkin pie, although bursting, consumed the second dinner to the last cranberry to oblige the first man. Both required hospitalization.

O. Henry's turn-of-the-century tales, *The Four Million* and *Sixes and Sevens,* dealt with the quest for nourishment (of all kinds). Our story, *The Rules of Tens and Twelves,* is a latter-day tale of nutrition.

The Rule of Tens (4 + 6) For Women	Food	The Rule of Twelves (5 + 7) For Men
Centicals		Centicals
4	Fruits	5
6	Vegetables	7
4	Milk and Meat	5
6	Grains	7

This chart gives a nutritionally balanced selection of foods for good health, cancer prevention, cardiovascular protection, and weight control. It will satisfy those who count calories, measure grams, or value vitamins.

We are now ready to structure our daily diet by selecting foods from the basic groups according to their *centical* content. The chart numbers refer to a unit of measurement I have dubbed the *centical*. You will find the amounts of different foods equivalent to one centical in the tables a few pages on in this chapter, but don't skip ahead to look just yet.

One centical equals 100 calories, more or less, or food providing 100 calories. It is not crucial that each food unit consumed be precisely 100 calories. Portions vary, and it is inconvenient and unnecessary to carry around a metric scale to weigh food, or a book of tables to look up its caloric content. Variations in caloric content of a food unit above or below an exact centical will tend to average out, even a 10 percent variation from one day to the next will average out. For example, if an average woman requires about 2,000 calories per day for normal internal metabolic energy requirements and average physical activity, she might range from 1,800 to 2,200 calories or 18 to 22 centicals in any given day, with day by day variations averaging out over the course of a typical week. Even a persistent 200 calorie error per day would, in the course of a week, result in only a 1,400 calorie gain or loss, which represents only 0.4 of a pound, an imperceptible change on the average home bathroom scale. For an average male requiring about 2,500 calories, a daily calorie range of 2,300 to 2,700 is acceptable. A needless pursuit of exact 100 calorie equivalents or any other measure will not improve any diet. It is the year-in, year-out structure of food consumption, not the daily variations, that matters.

The First Rule of Tens for Women

Women will consume 4 centicals (400 calories) of fruits per day, which will be derived from four selections of fruits, each more or less 100 calories energy equivalent. An adult woman will consume six portions of vegetables, each of 1 centical or 100 calorie energy content, for a total of 600 calories derived from vegetables. For milk and meat there will be four selections with a caloric value of 4 centicals or 400 calories and for grains, six selections with a caloric value of 6 centicals or 600 calories. Taken together these will yield approximately 2,000 calories per day, or somewhat less, because the vegetable units average less than 100 calories per piece.

The First Rule of Twelves for Men

In the same way men will use five and seven instead of four and six to determine the numbers of selections of foods to supply an adult male with about 2,400 calories per day.

The caloric intake range on a typical day is from 1,800 to 2,200 calories for a woman and from 2,200 to 2,600 calories for a man. The equilibrium between calories consumed in food and calories expended for metabolic and energy requirements varies from person to person depending on weight, physical activity, state of health, and environmental factors, such as climate. We maintain more or less stable weight most of the time without consciously making an effort to do so. An automatic governor within us seems to keep the energy out and in flowing with equal force. The meter runs all the time but at the end of the week, despite some variations from day to day, the figures read about the same.

As a rule of thumb you can calculate the number of calories you need per day to maintain your present weight by multiplying your weight by 15. For example, a 166 pound man will require 2,500 calories, assuming normal health and average physical activity. High fever, an overactive thyroid gland, or strenuous physical exertion will require higher caloric intake to maintain a steady state. For a woman weighing 133 pounds the daily steady-state calorie requirement is 133×15 or 2,000 calories. By decreasing your caloric intake by 500 to 1,000 calories per day, you will lose one to two pounds per week. A total daily caloric intake below 1,000 calories is not recommended. Weigh yourself one to three times a week to follow your progress. Keep a written record if you are trying to lose weight.

Begin by following the rule of tens and twelves. Your body's inner sense will tell you of the need to adjust upward or downward as energy needs vary.

For those having greater or lesser caloric needs and especially for those who wish to take off or put on weight, the rule of tens and twelves allows all the flexibility you need. Caloric changes of only 100 to 200 calories per day are not very meaningful; the diet may vary that much from day to day anyway. To increase or decrease food and calorie intake enough to matter, add or subtract one selection from each of the four food groups: fruits, vegetables, grains, and milk and meat. That will change your total caloric intake by 4 centicals (400 calories) per day. If this change is made not in response to a different caloric demand (strenuous or sedentary lifestyle) but in an attempt to lose or gain weight, 400 calories per day will cause a net true weight change of 0.8 pounds per week (500 calories per day change equals one pound per week weight change).

Thus a 133 pound woman who is at a metabolic steady state at a 2,000 calorie intake can lose 0.8 pounds per week by reducing her daily food intake by one *Optional Unit* containing one selection each of a fruit, vegetable, grain, and milk and meat—from a 4–6–4–6 pattern to a 3–5–3–5 pattern (1,600 calories per day). With a second optional unit reduction, she could reduce her caloric intake to 1,200 calories per day with an expected loss of 1.6 pounds per week. Caloric intake of less than 1,000 calories per day or weight loss of more than 2 pounds per week for long periods of time are not recommended. A male with average physical activity and weighing 166 pounds will require about 2,500 calories per day (166 × 15). Should he wish to gain weight or be involved in strenuous physical activity requiring higher caloric expenditure, he can simply add optional units containing one selection from each of the four categories, and thus go stepwise from 2,500 calories to 2,900, 3,300, and so on.

The division of our total food intake each day into more or less equal meal portions, spaced at conventional intervals, with or without between-meal snacks, is important. Snacks are a matter of personal preference as long as they are taken from the overall daily food allotment. Midmorning, midafternoon, and bedtime snacks are allowable. When optional units are added to or subtracted from the basic rule of tens and twelves, the optional unit should be spread throughout the day. For example, if you are adding an optional unit of one fruit, one vegetable, one grain, and one milk and meat, you might add the additional fruit to breakfast, the additional vegetable to lunch, the additional milk and meat to supper, and the additional grain to a bedtime snack.

To review before we go on: One centical equals about 100 calories. An adult woman of normal weight and average physical activity might require 18 to 22 centicals (1,800 to 2,200 calories) per day, a male 22 to 26 centicals (2,200 to 2,600 calories) per day. Variations depend on physical activity and whether weight change is desired. The number of selections (servings or portions) of food per day follows the rule of tens in women and the rule of twelves in men, apportioned among the four basic food categories of fruits, vegetables, grains, meat and milk, and divided 4–6–4–6 for women and 5–7–5–7 for men. An optional unit equivalent to 4 centicals (400 calories) per day equals one selection each from fruits, vegetables, grains, and milk and meat.

The Cafeteria Scoop
for Vegetables

People's idea of what constitutes a reasonable portion may vary, not to mention the differences in serving size between eating at home, a steak and potatoes restaurant, or a tea and sandwich parlor. For practical purposes the American cafeteria scoop is standard enough in size. Hairline precision is not crucial in our food measurements. For foods that lend themselves to scooping, a typical cafeteria will probably deposit 3 to 4 ounces on your plate, with 3 or 4 such portions comfortably occupying an ordinary dinner plate.

The centical (100 calorie) selection size works well for typical portions of most vegetables, with some rounding off for simplicity. When the cafeteria scoop is specified, you are being shortchanged a bit on your centical, but to no harm. It will not upset your calorie balance significantly with normal or even high vegetable consumption and allows a little leeway for the occasional indiscretion.

The Beta Unit

What is a beta unit? How many do you need per day? What is your margin for error? What is the evidence collected in the lab or from epidemiology studies to support the beta unit concept? Does cooking affect beta units?

A beta unit is an unscientific, accurate if not precise measurement of the cancer-blocking content in one portion of food. "Accurate but not precise" means that the concept is correct, and it matters little whether you consume 100 grams or only 99.99. The evidence is derived from studies on tissue cultures, laboratory animals, and from epidemiology studies of human populations around the world with low and high cancer rates. One beta unit per day is apparently sufficient to afford a high degree of protection against cancer. To be on the safe side I recommend two units per day. Averaging less than one beta unit per day is taking an unnecessary risk. We have no evidence that taking more than two beta units per day benefits cancer prevention. A beta unit provides one unit of cancer protection (whether beta-carotene or other active agent) and is found in one cafeteria scoop of the beta-carotene-containing foods:

Dark green, leafy vegetables such as spinach.

Dark yellow vegetables such as carrots.

Cruciferous vegetables, including cabbage, cauliflower, broccoli, and brussels sprouts.

The One-Centical Selection

A list of what constitutes a one-centical selection follows for your reference and curiosity, but it is not meant to be used as a continuing crutch. You will find the concept is easily learned and familiarity with the diet achieved.

In general, a centical is equivalent to:

Fruits: one piece of fruit or 6–8 oz. of juice.

Grains: 2 thin slices of bread, 1 cup (8 oz.) of cereal, or ½ cup of pasta.

Milk and Meat: 8 oz. skim milk, about a cafeteria scoop of chicken (3 oz.) or about ¼ to ⅓ of a fast-food-chain hamburger (about 1 oz. of meat).

Beta-carotene and Other Vegetables: The calorie count of a cafeteria scoop of beta-carotene or other vegetables is less than 50 calories, so a centical serving would be two cafeteria scoops, more than most people want to eat of one vegetable at a sitting. So each one cafeteria scoop vegetable selection will shortchange you, but the caloric undercount has negligible impact on the total diet plan, and in fact allows some leeway for modest cheating.

Legumes—peas and beans: one cafeteria scoop.

Nuts and Seeds: ½ oz.—about what you can get out of the package with a hefty scoop of a soup spoon.

To recapitulate, the typical portion, serving, or selection in each of the four main food categories produces one centical of energy equivalent. The number of selections from each food group is indicated in the chart at the beginning of this chapter.

The Second Rule of Tens and Twelves

To govern reshuffling centicals from the four food groups into convenient meals we invoke the Second Rule of Tens and Twelves: four and six for women, five and seven for men. The Master Plan Menu (Chapter 16) will clarify this.

For women:
breakfast—4 centicals
lunch—6 centicals
snacks—4 centicals (midmorning, midafternoon, and evening/bedtime)
supper—6 centicals

For men:
breakfast—5 centicals
lunch—7 centicals
snacks—5 centicals (midmorning, midafternoon, and evening/bedtime)
supper—7 centicals

For an individual taking part of a daily diet as snacks, the division of food units is shown in the Master Plan Menu. For women, for example, breakfast consists of 4 centical units, preferably one from each of the four food groups; lunch, 6 units selected from among the four food groups; and so on. Snack units may be divided among 1, 2, or 3 snack periods or, if no snack periods are elected, then the 4 units can be more or less evenly distributed among the three regular meals. The division of the daily food supply into meals selected from the four food groups will be shown in detail in Chapter 16.

The Food List

Centical size portions are indicated. Food weights are for the usual edible parts:

Vegetables and fruits: carrot greens (sprigs) removed; broccoli stalks cut short; peas and beans shelled; all vegetables cleaned and trimmed; nuts and seeds hulled and shelled; inedible pits, seeds, rinds, stems and stalks removed; bananas skinned; and oranges peeled.

Whole grains are preferrred.

Fat-free milk and dairy products are indicated. Trim fat, leaving meat as lean as possible; skin chicken and turkey. Shellfish meats are weighed without shells.

GROUP A
Vegetables

	Weight in oz.	Calories
1. *Beta-carotene vegetables* (one cafeteria scoop)		
Spinach	4	29
Carrots	4	39
Cabbage	4	21
Broccoli	4	28
Cauliflower	4	30
Brussels sprouts	4	47
2. *Legumes* (one cafeteria scoop)		
Peas	4	95
Beans (lima)	4	139
Beans (green)	4	32
3. *Nuts and Seeds* (one heaping soup spoon)		
Soy nuts	½	57
Sunflower seeds	½	79
Peanuts	½	80
Pecans	½	96
Almonds	½	102
Walnuts	½	90

	Weight in oz.	Calories
4. *Other Vegetables* (one cafeteria scoop)		
Asparagus	4	16
Beets	4	34
Celery	4	14
Cucumbers	4	16
Eggplant	4	23
Lettuce	4	11
Mushrooms	4	31
Onions	4	39
Peppers	4	20
Radishes	4	17
Squash (summer)	4	22
Squash (winter)	4	38
Tomatoes	4	25
Turnips	4	29

GROUP B
Fruits

	One Centical (100 calories) (*Note:* 1 cup = 8 oz.)
Apples	1 medium or 6 oz. juice
Apricots	6 medium
Bananas	1 medium
Berries	½ lb.
Canteloupes	1 medium
Cherries	½ lb.
Dates and Figs	2 medium
Grapefruits	1 small or 8 oz. juice
Grapes	50, or 4 oz. juice
Lemons	5 average
Oranges	2 medium or 8 oz. juice
Peaches	3 medium
Pears	1 average

	One Centical (100 calories) (Note: 1 cup = 8 oz.)
Pineapples	½ lb. or 5 oz. juice
Plums	15 small
Prunes	5 large or 4 oz. juice
Raisins	1 oz.
Watermelons	1 large slice

GROUP C
Grains and Cereals (and starchy vegetables)

	One Centical (100 calories)
Bread	1½–2 slices
Crackers	5 to 10 (approx.)
Pancakes	2
Waffles	1
Cornflakes or Rice Krispies	1 cup (8 oz.)
Potatoes	1 large (6 oz.)
Rice	½ cup
Pizza	⅛ medium-size pizza
Ravioli	4 oz.
Noodles	½ cup
Spaghetti	½ cup

GROUP D
Milk, Meat, Poultry, and Fish

	One Centical (100 Calories)
	Oz.
Skim milk	8 (1 cup)
Meats	
Hamburger or Steak	1 (approx.—depends on % of fat)
Veal	1½
Poultry	
Chicken	3–4
Turkey	2
Fish	
Cod, Sole, Trout, Bass, Swordfish, etc.	4
Tuna (canned in water)	3–4

	Oz.
Shellfish	
Lobster tail	1 tail
Shrimp	4
Clams	16 (2 cups)
Scallops	4
Cottage cheese	
Uncreamed, low fat	4

Summation

A diet of such composition will be well balanced in terms of grams of fat, carbohydrate, and protein; will have appropriate limitation of saturated animal fat and cholesterol; should not provide excessive quantities of sugar or salt; and will contain sufficient vitamins and minerals for the nutrition of normal adult men and women.

The beta-carotene diet initial test period consists of the first week, during which minor adjustments in portion size may be made in response to differences in metabolic rates, physical activity, and moderated (but not dominated) by your feelings of hunger or satiation.

It is simple to model the diet to your particular needs depending on your age, sex, metabolic rate, physical activity, and desire to lose or gain weight, by adding or subtracting an Optional Unit of 4 centicals (400 calories): one fruit unit, one vegetable unit, one milk and meat unit, and one grain unit. Let us assume that you wish to lose weight and that you are female. According to the First Rule of Tens your food units are distributed between the four primary food groups: 4–6–4–6. Subtracting one food unit from each leaves 3–5–3–5. This plan will maintain a reasonable balance between the food groups consumed and the relative numbers of grams of fat, protein, carbohydrate, and other nutrients, and will decrease your caloric intake by about 400 calories per day, from approximately 2,000 to 1,600 calories. Over the course of a week this will yield a net deficit of 2,800 calories below the number necessary to maintain you in a steady state of weight, that is, 2,800 calories less than you consume for internal metabolic energy requirements and for external physical activity. With 3,500 calories equal to one pound, your net weight loss for the week will be 0.8 true pounds.

By reducing your food intake by two optional units you will reduce your calorie consumption by 800 calories per day, which works out to a weight loss of 1.6 true pounds per week. One to two pounds of weight loss per week and a minimum caloric intake of 1,000 calories is recommended for both men and women.

The division of total food intake per day into a meal plan consistent with cultural, work and school, and social patterns is important. In addition, consuming most daily food at a single sitting unnecessarily stresses digestion and the metabolic processing of the food, producing undesirable temporary high blood levels of sugar and fat.

Division of daily food into three meals with no snacks or up to three snacks (midmorning, midafternoon, and/or evening or bedtime) is advised, according to the Second Rule of Tens (for women) and Twelves (for men).

Don't forget your daily beta units. One to two beta units per day are apparently sufficient—more do not appear to be any more effective. The cancer-blocking agent apparently operates by interfering with or blocking the promotion stage of cancer rather than the initiation, hence its value if started anytime in life. Although cooking does not appear to affect the beta unit protection, at least one of the two units per day should probably be from fresh food, not canned or frozen, served uncooked.

Have you had your beta unit today?

FIFTEEN

QUESTIONS AND ANSWERS

I want to lose weight. Every diet I try works for a while but I can't seem to stick with it long enough. What can I do?

The beta-carotene diet has certain advantages. Anyone would tire of a perpetual grapefruit diet, begin to feel self-conscious about the foul breath associated with ketotic diets, or get worried when they read in the newspapers about diets causing dangerously low potassium levels. Pep talks about motivation or the psychological reasons people overeat only increase our anxiety levels.

The beta-carotene diet, because it is a diet structured for permanence, resembles old-fashioned eating habits in many ways and serves many purposes: heart disease and cancer prevention; high blood pressure, diabetes, and obesity protection; as well as the cosmetic aspects of weight loss. It is easy to follow and gives you a subtle, even smug, feeling that you've taken yourself in hand and are really doing something at last.

What about people who hate vegetables?

Most of us can relearn our eating habits, which were established in early childhood and are largely cultural, not intrinsic.

Vegetables can be prepared in dozens of ways with their appearance and taste varied and attractive.

What about people with diabetes, arteriosclerosis, high blood pressure, or diverticulosis?

The diet is low in sugar, cholesterol and animal fat, and salt. It should be compatible with most special dietary and medication needs. All persons, under treatment or not, should check with their physicians before altering diet. Diverticulosis has traditionally been treated with low fiber (low residue) diets but that is now controversial. People on high fiber diets do not get diverticulosis. The objectives of the beta-carotene diet can be achieved by limiting other vegetables and whole grains in patients with established diverticulosis, if bowel symptoms occur with high fiber.

Does food preparation matter?

Epidemiology data from around the world do not show any difference in anticancer effect from the method of food preparation or preservation. Foods may be fresh, canned, or frozen and may be eaten raw or cooked. We do know that long storage of food or prolonged high cooking temperature does affect many biochemical substances and organic nutrients. So it would appear prudent not to subject beta-carotene foods to such treatment and to eat one fresh, uncooked beta-carotene food daily.

I've never been able to stay on any diet for long. Can I achieve the cancer protection effect without strict adherence to the entire diet?

Yes. In a nutshell, decrease your intake of animal fat and be sure to have at least one or two beta units per day. Stay thin, don't smoke, and drink little, if at all.

What about foods not on the list?

Use common sense and your knowledge to assign unlisted foods to the proper food category. In any case, occasional lapses or variations from the overall diet are unimportant.

What if I go off the diet for a few days and go on vacation and eat everything for two weeks?

The diet is not a rigid prescription; you can deviate from it and substitute reasonably. You can even go off it for short periods. Eating is a pleasure. We can condition ourselves to find that pleasure in beneficial foods, creatively prepared and served. For those of us with certain lifelong food preferences, occasional lapses are not harmful. Munching on broccoli stalks at a testimonial dinner honoring your 25 years of service to the company while everyone else is dining on lobster tail and roast beef is sure to make you feel miserable.

Can this diet be used just for temporary purposes to help lose weight?

The beta-carotene diet is not intended as a temporary crash diet plan nor will it serve that purpose. It is meant as a lifetime eating formula, in many ways not very different from what you may have been eating all along, but with the crucial changes noted.

Will the diet help after cancer has been diagnosed?

For a clinically diagnosed cancer there are no data showing any significant benefit. We do know that at the cellular level, early changes in the development of cancer can be reversed by retinoids (synthetic Vitamin A-like compounds).

I'm a vegetarian. Can I use the diet?

Yes. For vegetarians who do not eat red meats but will eat chicken or fish, no modification of the beta-carotene diet is needed. Adaptation is required to furnish adequate protein for more restrictive vegetarians.

Lacto-ovo-vegetarians do not consume red meat, chicken or fish, but do use dairy products and eggs, sources of ample protein. Choice of skim milk products and egg whites whenever milk or meat is called for works nicely. Lactovegetarians follow the same practices but exclude eggs—no problem, either.

For pure vegetarians who consume foods solely of plant origin, protein needs can be met, but it takes a little planning.

Animal proteins contain all the essential amino acids we need in sufficient quantity and proportion. Plant proteins from any single plant source are deficient in one or another of the amino acids humans require to synthesize human protein, but by combining plant sources at the same meal the whole spectrum of amino acids is easily obtained. Whole grain products contain most of the amino acids. By eating any vegetable (including legumes, nuts, and seeds) at the same sitting, the needed balance of amino acids is met.

Pure vegetarians may need a supplement of Vitamin B_{12}, which is not abundant in plant sources. Some soybean milk is fortified with Vitamin B_{12}. Pure vegetarians also need ample whole grains for riboflavin, dark green vegetables and nuts for calcium, and enriched grain sources for iron.

SIXTEEN

THE MASTER PLAN
FOR YOUR
DAILY MENU

On the following pages is a simple, brief master plan for your daily menu, incorporating the anticancer weight-control principles outlined in the chapters you have just read.

1. Any recipe consistent with the beta-carotene diet plan can be used, and almost every recipe can be adapted.

2. Consider rich sauces and gravies, butter, heavy cream, and egg yolks unfit for human consumption. Get to know and enjoy the natural flavor, aroma, and eye appeal of the almost infinite variety of available foods.

3. The diet is meant to be flexible. As long as the basic principles are observed, you can vary it to your own schedule or habits, food preferences, spices, and seasonal availability of foods.

4. You can substitute foods not on the list according to your common-sense understanding of their food grouping and appropriateness.

5. Individuals with diabetes, high blood pressure, diverticulosis, and more, can easily adapt the beta-carotene diet to their needs. A physician should be consulted for assistance.

6. Persons contemplating a change in lifestyle, be it weight loss,

change in diet, an exercise program, or a trip to the tropics, would be wise to consult their doctors.

7. Food portions or quantities on the master menu are as indicated on the lists in Chapter 14, and contain approximately 100 calories. Especially for vegetables it is less, so the diet as written delivers somewhat fewer calories than the theoretical number of 2,000 (women) or 2,400 (men). That does not concern us at all. Your sense of fullness after eating and your bathroom scale will guide adjustments in food consumption.

8. Particularly for women who want to lose weight now, the diet may seem too generous. You do not have to clean your plate! Decrease from 2,000 to 1,600 calories by omitting an Optional Unit (one fruit, one vegetable, one grain, and one milk or meat) per day. Decrease to 1,200 calories by omitting a second Optional Unit.

9. You may want to use the Snack Option by saving a food selection from a meal for later in the day.

10. Men doing heavy work can meet energy needs by adding Optional Units.

Sample Daily Menu Master Plan*

Meal	Food Group	No. of 100-Calorie Portions Women	Men	Women	For Men Add:
Breakfast	Fruits	1	2	orange or other fruit juice	banana or berries (in cereal if you wish)
	Vegetables	1	1	sunflower seeds (sprinkle on cereal)	
	Milk/Meat	1	1	skim milk (as drink, in cereal, in coffee)	
	Grains	2	2	bran or other cereal; whole wheat or other toast	

Midmorning snack if desired: any unused breakfast portions

| Meal | Food Group | No. of 100-Calorie Portions | | Women | For Men Add: |
		Women	Men		
Lunch	Fruits	2	2	large apple, peach, or cluster of grapes (double portion)	
	Vegetables	2	3	tomato slices and/or lettuce, fresh raw broccoli, cauliflower tips or shredded cabbage	fresh green peas or soy nuts
	Milk/Meat	1	1	tunafish, lowfat cheese, or uncreamed, lowfat cottage cheese	
	Grains	2	3	hard roll, rye, or other bread, biscuits, muffins, or crackers (double portion)	rice, corn, or potato

Midafternoon snack if desired: any unused lunch portions

Dinner	Fruits	1	1	grapefruit or cantaloupe	
	Vegetables	3	3	spinach salad, carrots or other beta-carotene vegetable; green beans or any other vegetable	
	Milk/Meat	2	3	chicken or fish, uncreamed lowfat cottage cheese or skim milk (double portion)	additional serving
	Grains	2	2	any pasta, rice, corn, potato, or bread (double portion)	

Evening snack if desired: any unused dinner portions

*See lists in Chapter 14 for portion sizes.

SEVENTEEN

BETA-CAROTENE RECIPES

Main Courses

Be creative and remember that chicken, veal, or fish combined in any butterless way with the Big Six beta-carotene vegetables (Group A1) add up to a weight loss and cancer prevention program. The variations are limitless and happily habit-forming. You will soon lose your craving for the things you know are bad for you.

Chicken and Broccoli Casserole

Note: It is always best to buy boneless breast of chicken. The pennies per pound lower price of whole chickens is a deception, because with cheaper cuts you are paying for bone and *fat*—just what you do not want.

chicken, trimmed and cubed
corn, safflower, or sunflower oil/margarine (a little)
garlic
diced, sweet red pepper
canned, drained green peas
broccoli
white—or better—long-grained wild rice

In a wide skillet, sauté (stir-fry briefly over medium heat—always avoid prolonged high heat) cubed chicken in margarine until slightly browned. Add garlic, red pepper, green peas, and broccoli. Stir-fry in the vegetables. Prepare the rice in a separate skillet, following package directions. Let stand for seven or eight minutes. Now, European style, fold rice into the chicken and vegetable mixture. Serve fresh carrot sticks on the side, also, perhaps, shredded lettuce. The diced pepper makes this a real show-off casserole.

Chicken and Scallions

This recipe will change your approach to main course preparation. You may never use flour or cornstarch again. Apply the idea to all your cooking. Choice of ingredients and method of preparation are simple, without sacrificing eye and palate appeal.

chicken, diced and boned

corn, safflower, or sunflower oil/margarine (a little)

garlic

scallions, trimmed, diced (keep some green shoots aside)

eggs, 3 or so—*you* decide what you need.

Sauté (brief, low heat) chicken chunks in margarine and garlic. Toss in scallions, diced white circles first. Simmer. Separate egg yolks and whites, storing whites (the high-protein part) in a bowl. Put egg yolks where they belong—in the garbage.

Now for the magic part. Pour in liquid egg whites at medium heat and stir, stir, stir. Watch egg whites become your thickening agent. Add more garlic to taste and now add the green shoots from the tops of the scallions for color. Simmer.

Serve with rice and, of course, a side of broccoli or one of the other Big Six beta-carotene vegetables.

Side Dishes

Perhaps the Big Six beta-carotene anticancer vegetables are not your favorite vegetables (you would rather have sweet corn-on-the-cob), so the following recipes will teach you how to make them delicious and attractive. And you can have sweet corn, too.

Vegetables are best eaten raw, or undercooked in small quantities of water. When cooking oil is used it should be polyunsaturated (corn, sunflower, safflower), scant in quantity, and not subjected to prolonged high heat.

Spinach Ricotta (Beta-Carotene and Low-Cholesterol Style)

Note: The heavy creams, cheeses, and egg yolks of this recipe have been left in the supermarket.

diced onions

corn oil margarine (sparingly)

spinach (canned is acceptable)

tofu (Japanese ground soybeans)

nutmeg

In wide skillet, sauté diced onion in corn oil margarine until soft and brown. Drain spinach (if canned), add to onions, chop to avoid stringy look, and mix. Mash in tofu, lots of it. (Tofu is high in protein, low in everything you want it to be, and probably the food of the future. Get used to it.)

Now add the nutmeg. The aroma is gourmet, and the taste is so good!

Three-Vegetable Casserole

cauliflower

carrots

broccoli

corn oil margarine (sparingly)

thyme

For convenience, buy frozen, prepared bags of vegetables; or if you love chopping, make them fresh.

Combine vegetables with water in a deep cooker, bring to a boil, pour off water, and add margarine and thyme. Toss. Let sit a few minutes for aromas to mingle. Toss again. This is a colorful casserole, and is also good cold, as a summer side dish.

Needless to say, any of the Big Six beta-carotene vegetables can be served alone, boiled or sautéed a little, with a touch of margarine.

Spinach Salad

spinach, fresh
onions, chopped
croutons, spiced
1 tsp. corn oil
vinegar
garlic, basil, oregano to taste

Good with any main course.

THE
CANCER
AROUND
US

EIGHTEEN

CANCER SCIENCE: THE BACKGROUND

Extraordinary scientific works were published as we entered the 1980s. Their subject was cancer. They dovetail remarkably. In a moment you will be reading about their conclusions.

In scientific research, shared instincts and a common fund of knowledge often culminate in simultaneous discoveries, by researchers sometimes in concert, sometimes in conflict.

Especially now, when news dissemination is a matter of milliseconds, not months, why the man in the street and many professionals are unaware of the news about cancer is a mystery.

As you will see, what you did yesterday and the food you ate may have increased your chances of becoming a cancer statistic. After reading this chapter you will know how you can begin today to become, if not immune to, at least shielded from, unnecessary tumors.

This part of the book can be used as a reference. Just flip through or find what you want in the Index, whether it be selenium or zinc, Vitamin C, PCBs, or the geography of stomach cancer.

Background—Old and New

Many other causes of cancer have been identified since Sir Percival Pott in 1775 described the first environmental cancer, cancer of the scrotum in chimney sweeps: cigarettes and lung cancer, asbestos and mesothelioma, DES (diethylstilbestrol) and vaginal cancer in female offspring, and more.

Fat may influence the development of breast cancer by its effect on increasing estrogenic and pituitary hormones, and may influence colon cancer by increasing the flow of bile salts and their metabolites into the bowel.

In some but not all studies, very low cholesterol levels, under 180, seemed to correlate with higher cancer mortality. It is possible that low cholesterol does not cause cancer but is a result of the malignant process. Many such questions are raised in medicine as a result of observation in a handful of studies. Statistical correlation does not prove a cause-and-effect relationship. There is no cause at this time to diminish the efforts to reduce blood cholesterol in our population, especially because the benefit of reducing coronary artery disease is so great.

Evaluating all potential chemical carcinogens is virtually impossible. There are 4,000,000 existing chemicals, 60,000 in widespread use, and about 1,000 new ones each year.

Chemicals that are carcinogenic for humans include arsenic, asbestos, benzene, chromium, DES, soot and tars, and vinyl chloride; also aflatoxins, cadmium, nickel, carbon tetrachloride, phenacetin, and PCBs.

Initiating agents produce mutational changes in cells and some may cause carcinoma (cancer) in and of themselves. A single exposure may be sufficient and the effect is irreversible. Promoting agents must be given after an initiating agent—they are not carcinogenic alone. Prolonged exposure is required and, at an early stage, the action is reversible.

Scientists collect data about cancer and diet in three ways:

In the lab, the test-tube approach, tissue cultures are exposed to possible carcinogens—cancer-producing agents—after which the cells, chromosomes, and genes are studied for damage.

In animal laboratories, cancer vulnerability is measured against controlled variations in environment and food supply. Animal data may not reflect human biology.

Finally, people are studied—the most relevant but the most complex way to gather scientific information. Because of the difficulties in controlling any one factor in the lives of large numbers of people, data must be analyzed and conclusions drawn with care. Whether a study is retrospective (looking at the past) or prospective (trying to influence future behavior), proof requires two large groups of subjects, equivalent except for the factor under study. If more cancers arise in one group than the other, we have taken a step toward finding a cause-and-effect relationship.

When all three kinds of studies are in agreement, we can start to talk about clinical proof or proof for practical purposes. Absolute proof, when it comes to human biology, is unachievable for practical as well as moral and ethical considerations, but is not necessary, an issue we shall deal with in more detail.

There are ten trillion cells in each adult human body. The number of cell divisions occurring during a normal lifetime is staggering, equal to 1,000 times ten trillion. An aberration in a single cell during one cell division can result in a cancer. The relative infrequency of cancer gives testimony to the reliability of our biologic systems: the control mechanism that regulates cell reproduction and the immune mechanism that detects and destroys faulty cells. From the single cell formed at the moment of conception of a new human, many cells with different forms and functions will develop. Yet all must act in concert. It is awesome as we recognize that genetic and cellular defects as a rule arise from the environment, not from within. A considerable body of evidence supports this concept: cigarettes or asbestos and lung cancer, certain chemical dyes and bladder cancer, the change in cancer rates in groups migrating from one country to another; the evidence against the environment we live in and the food we eat cannot be ignored.

Earlier, we talked about the initiation, latent period (often long), and promotion of cancer, phases in the development of cancer. Dietary changes appear to affect the promotion of cancer, which is good news for most of us. Identifying and excluding initiator substances would help only the very young. For people who do not yet have cancer, a dietary change that interferes with promotion could be a lifetime shield against cancer.

Two million people in the United States will die this year. One out of every five of the deaths will be due to cancer. One out of every four people in the country will have cancer during his or her lifetime.

With the population of the United States now over two hundred million, that is more than 50 million cancers in Americans now living.

Before exploring cancer science, a word about cancer quackery. In *Laetrile in Historical Perspective* (*Connecticut Medicine*, August 1979), James Harvey Young, Ph.D., described the ten-point formula employed by health quacks to delude and exploit the public. The methods:

1. Fear.
2. Guarantees of cure without pain.
3. Claiming a miraculous new breakthrough.
4. Oversimplifying the nature of a disease and the solution to its treatment.
5. Asserting that, if not now, future scientists will applaud their theories.
6. Implying that professional antagonisms are the reasons for lack of current recognition.
7. Articulate and deceptive defenses of their position.
8. Citing individual case histories or glowing testimonials from believers as proof, overlooking misdiagnosis, spontaneous remission, and effects of legitimate treatment.
9. Invoking the patient's right to seek any so-called treatment.
10. The treatment is expensive and the profits are channeled directly to the proponents of the treatment.

By contrast, the scientific sources cited have impeccable credentials in cancer research:

1. *Diet, Nutrition, and Cancer,* The Committee on Diet, Nutrition, and Cancer of the National Research Council, 1982. Renowned and cautious scientists and professors from Yale, Harvard, the National Cancer Institute of Canada, the National Cancer Center Research Institute of Japan, and other centers brought a broad spectrum of medical expertise to sift and study the world literature (more than one thousand published papers) on cancer research and published their landmark conclusions in a report hundreds of pages long.

2. *Can Dietary Beta-Carotene Materially Reduce Human Cancer Rates?* The Imperial Cancer Research Fund Cancer Studies and Epidemiology Units, Great Britain, and the National Cancer Insti-

tute, Bethesda, Maryland, by Richard Peto, Richard Doll, et al., published in the leading scientific journal *Nature*, 1981, with ground breaking impact.

3. *The Causes of Cancer: Quantitative Estimates of Avoidable Risks of Cancer in the United States Today*, published in the *Journal of the National Cancer Institute* (National Institutes of Health), by Doll and Peto in 1981.

4. *Does Life Style Cause Cancer?* A symposium published in the *New York State Journal of Medicine* in 1980.

Let us look now at the scientific evidence: how our diet and environment provoke or prevent cancer.

NINETEEN

DIET, NUTRITION, AND CANCER

The report published in 1982 of the Committee on Diet, Nutrition, and Cancer of the National Research Council states that the overwhelming majority of human cancers are caused by the environment and are potentially preventable. Cancer is not a predestined genetic fact of life. Our air, water, food, where we live, and the work we do correlate with cancers of the gastrointestinal tract, lungs, urinary tract, and reproductive organs. The nature of such relationships is becoming clear to scientists and should become common knowledge to the public, as familiar as the diet for the prevention of heart disease became in the 1970s.

The following are some of the factors we will look at in detail.

1. *Total caloric intake:* Less food correlates with less cancer and longer lifespan, obesity and high-calorie intake with more cancer.

2. *Fats (lipids),* especially fat of animal origin, or saturated fat: Cancers of the breast, colon, and prostate appear to be related to the amount of fat in the diet. A relationship between cholesterol and cancer is not clear, although some studies suggest that an uncommonly low cholesterol level correlates with increased colon cancer. This remains far from proven and should not discourage anyone from following a low-cholesterol diet now.

3. *Protein:* Excessive protein intake may correlate with cancer, but foods high in protein often contain fat as well, and an independent effect of protein is uncertain.

4. *Carbohydrates:* There is no data implicating carbohydrates, aside from their relationship to caloric intake, but a few studies relate high sugar or starch intake to certain tumors.

5. *Fiber:* This refers to indigestible substances in food generally associated with carbohydrates, such as cellulose, lignins, and pectin. These are common in grains, fruits, and vegetables and provide bulk in the diet.

High fiber may have a beneficial effect in protecting against colon cancer by its bulk. It induces more rapid transit through the large bowel and earlier bowel movements, thereby decreasing the time during which potential carcinogens in the fecal stream are in contact with the bowel wall. Other mechanisms are also possible. Different types of fiber are under study, as well as total fiber content.

6. *Vitamin A (retinol)* and its precursors, the carotenoids: These may inhibit cancers at some sites. Synthetic analogs (retinoids) appear to inhibit cancers of the lung, bladder, and breast. Carotenoids are found in dark green or deep yellow vegetables, cabbage, broccoli, cauliflower, and brussels sprouts. Whether the inhibitor is Vitamin A, carotene, or some substance yet to be identified in these foods, is unclear.

7. *Vitamin C (ascorbic acid):* Foods containing Vitamin C may have a beneficial effect in lowering the risk of stomach and esophageal cancer. Ascorbic acid blocks the production of certain cancer-causing substances (*N*-nitroso compounds). Vitamin C is found in citrus fruits. The amount needed is controversial.

8. *Vitamin E (alphatocopherol):* This vitamin occurs in many foods, especially cereals and vegetables. It also blocks the chemical production of nitrosamines. The amount needed is controversial.

9. *B vitamins* are not clearly related to cancer.

10. *Minerals:* Selenium may be protective against cancer but the evidence is scanty. Low iron states may be related to cancer of the upper gastrointestinal tract. The National Research Council Commit-

tee also examined the evidence relating to copper, iodine, molybdenum, and zinc and could not conclude from available data any clearcut relationships for or against cancer. In the case of arsenic, cadmium, and lead, studies were likewise inconclusive, although there have been occasional case reports linking all these minerals with or against cancers. Occupational exposure to some minerals increases cancer risk.

11. *Alcohol:* Alcohol may be responsible for increased risk of various gastrointestinal cancers, such as liver and colon. In combination with smoking, alcohol may increase head, neck, and esophageal tumors.

12. *Nonnutritive Substances:* In addition to nutrients, food that has some value or use in human biology, there are nonnutritive substances, hitchhikers in food, that can stimulate cancer. The best known compounds in this category are the mycotoxins, particularly aflatoxin in peanut butter, and hydrazines in mushrooms.

13. *Mutagens and Flavonoids:* These are substances that affect genes, acting as initators of the cancer process. Some mutagens are produced by charcoal broiling or smoking of foods, benzo(a)pyrene, for example, or by cooking fish or meat at very high temperatures. Flavonoids are found in some vegetables.

14. *Food Additives and Contaminants:* An extraordinary number of substances are added to foods in America and an even greater number of other materials are used for food packaging and may find their way into food. In food processing, 3,000 compounds are added and 12,000 are used in packaging. Saccharin is an example of a food additive with known carcinogenic effect on laboratory animals. Vinyl chloride is known to be a cancer-producing agent in humans and has been used for food packaging.

Pesticides used in agriculture and the chemical waste products of American industry, such as polychlorinated biphenyls, find their way into the food chain.

15. *Epidemiology:* A geographical study of human disease patterns, one of our best clues for understanding and combatting cancer.

Some authorities conclude that up to 90 percent of human cancers are the result of environmental factors, including the food we eat. For women 60 percent of cancers and for men 40 percent of cancers are attributed to diet. The gastrointestinal system, lungs, and reproductive organs are most affected and would most benefit from changes.

It would seem prudent to make changes in our diet consistent with what we know about the diet–cancer equation, providing that the diet is nutritional; not in conflict with the dietary management of cardiovascular disease, diabetes, and hypertension; and that we know of no risks.

The National Research Council Committee on Diet, Nutrition, and Cancer recommendations:

Major Emphasis

1. Decrease fat, both saturated and unsaturated, from 40 to 30 percent or less of total calories, to decrease breast and colon cancers.

2. Include grain products, vegetables, and fruits in the diet, especially citrus fruits and the carotene-containing vegetables noted above. Since the anticancer relationship has been established with the foods themselves rather than with purified concentrates of individual substances such as Vitamin A, it would appear premature and possibly dangerous to use large quantities of such vitamins, and may miss the mark if the anticancer effect resides in some unidentified substance in those foods in which Vitamin A is only coincidentally present.

3. Smoked, salt-cured, and pickled foods correlate with an increased rate of upper gastrointestinal, esophageal, and stomach cancers. Such processing may produce carcinogenic effects by increasing the amount of N-nitroso compounds and polycyclic aromatic hydrocarbons.

4. Nonnutritive substances without any value, some of which occur naturally in foods, others added during food processing intentionally or unintentionally, should be eliminated from food as much as possible.

5. Alcohol consumption and cigarette smoking cause cancer in the head and neck, gastrointestinal tract, and respiratory organs. To-

gether the cancer stimulus is greater than by using either alone. Heavy beer drinking appears to be related to rectal cancer in the United States. Prolonged high alcohol ingestion with liver damage and cirrhosis may precede the development of a hepatoma, a cancer of the liver.

Vitamins

Vitamin A (retinol): Much of the research on Vitamin A has been in green and yellow vegetables having a high beta-carotene content, a Vitamin A precursor that is converted by the body into Vitamin A. A high intake of these foods correlates with lower occurrence of lung, laryngeal, esophageal, stomach, colon, bladder, and prostate cancer. There appears to be a general relationship between high intake of Vitamin A and beta-carotene foods and low incidence of cancer. But excessive amounts of Vitamin A can be toxic. We consider the class of foods, not Vitamin A nor beta-carotene, to be anticancer.

Synthetic compounds called *retinoids*, chemically related to Vitamin A, are being studied for possible antitumor effect. Retinoids do not occur normally in food. Beta-carotene is itself a member of a group of substances called *carotenoids*, which are under study. Vitamin A is found in whole milk and in liver, and beta-carotene in dark green and deep yellow vegetables.

Without Vitamin A the cell lining (epithelium) of many organs may not form normally, resulting in *metaplasia*, a cell change with the potential for cancer. Vitamin A may prevent the metaplasia induced by tumor-causing chemicals.

The daily requirement of Vitamin A is 5,000 IU. Doses of 50,000 IU per day over a period of several months is toxic.

Vitamin C (ascorbic acid): Studies of Vitamin C are most often studies on foods high in Vitamin C. A lower rate of cancer of the stomach and the esophagus is associated with consumption of citrus fruits. Vitamin C prevents the conversion of nitrites to nitroso compounds which are carcinogenic.

The daily requirement of 60 mg. is easily met by diets containing citrus fruits or cruciferous vegetables. The value of mega-doses of Vitamin C is controversial at best.

Vitamin E (alphatocopherol): Vitamin E occurs in many foods,

112

particularly grain products and vegetables, and also in eggs. Like Vitamin C, Vitamin E blocks the formation of nitroso compounds. In theory, this decreases esophageal and stomach cancer but there are no definite human studies.

B vitamins and *Vitamin D* do not have a known relationship to cancer causation or prevention.

Minerals

Selenium: Selenium deficiency may correlate with a higher incidence of cancer of many organs, including the colon and pancreas, lung, female reproductive organs, and bladder. Selenium is found in drinking water, seafood, meat, and cereal. The amount needed daily (50–200 one-millionths of a gram) is easily supplied by a normal diet. However, increasing the daily amount of selenium consumed to high levels in supplement form does not produce any benefits beyond that of a normal diet. Large amounts are toxic.

Zinc: Zinc is a component of a large number of human enzyme systems. A clearcut relationship to cancer, however, is not at present evident. Both high levels and low levels of zinc have been reported in association with tumors.

Iron: Iron deficiency correlates with increased cancer of the esophagus and stomach.

Copper: A clearcut relationship with cancer has not been identified.

Iodine: Where the iodine content of food and water is low there is an increase in goiter, a benign thyroid growth. Thyroid cancer may also increase in low-iodine areas.

Molybdenum: A possible relationship between low molybdenum levels and cancer of the esophagus in China and Africa has been reported, but definite evidence is lacking.

Cadmium: Kidney and prostate cancer may be associated with occupational exposure to cadmium but dietary consumption of cadmium has caused mixed results in different studies. Cadmium is a component of cigarette smoke.

Arsenic: Occupational exposure to arsenic (inhalation) correlates with lung cancer. Arsenic in food or water is not a proven cause of cancer, except possibly skin cancer.

Lead: Lead is found in various sources, such as automobile exhausts, paint, food, and water. Animal experiments suggest a possible cancer-causing effect but there is no direct confirmation in humans.

Nonnutritive Substances Found in Food

Food Additives and Contaminants

Food additives are substances that are intentionally added to food, almost 3,000 in number at present, about half of which are flavoring agents and 30 of which are coloring agents. About 500 to 600 are substances generally regarded as safe, such as spices and seasonings; another 500 or so are preservatives, stabilizers, leavening agents, antioxidants, emulsifiers, and sweeteners.

About 12,000 additional substances contaminate the food we eat. Any chemical used in the cleaning or operation of food processing machinery or in packaging materials may enter the food. Pesticides used on crops, bacteria, and fungi, and drugs given to animals may also become food contaminants.

So along with the protein, fat, carbohydrate, vitamins, and minerals in food, a large number of other substances are consumed. Very little is known about most of the nonnutritive substances, their effect on human biology or on cancer.

Food additives that are suspected carcinogens in animals include:

Cyclamates: Nonnutritive sweetener; bladder cancer in rats.

Saccharin: Nonnutritive sweetener; bladder cancer in several species of animals.

Sucrose: Sweetener; liver cancer in female mice.

FD&C (Food, Drug, and Cosmetic) Red #32: Food color; lung and breast cancer in mice.

FD&C Orange #2: Food color; intestinal cancer in mice.

Less familiar sounding agents on the list (flavoring agents, preservatives, antioxidants, extractants, emulsifiers, and stabilizers) cause a variety of tumors, mostly gastrointestinal, including liver, lung, and bladder cancer in rats and mice. With the exception of saccharin these additives are banned in human foods.

Contaminants include:

114

Polyvinyl chloride (PVC): found in packaging material.

DES (diethylstilbestrol): a female synthetic hormone fed to some animals.

Pesticides and parathion: enter the food cycle when contaminated plants are fed to animals.

PAHs (polycyclic aromatic hydrocarbons): for example, benzo(a)pyrene, from air pollution or charcoal broiling.

PCBs (polychlorinated biphenyls): found in freshwater fish and packaging materials.

Naturally occurring carcinogens:

Aflatoxin (a mycotoxin, fungal derivative): found in mold on peanuts and peanut butter.

Nitrosamines: derived from nitrites and amines in foods, which produce tumors in numerous organs: the liver, bladder, kidneys, stomach, intestines, and adrenal glands. Mice and rats are the primary test species. Nitrates and nitrites are widely used as meat product preservatives. Nitrate converts readily to nitrite, which in combination with amines or amides in food produces N-nitroso compounds. Such compounds are clearly carcinogenic in animal species and probably cause human cancers of the esophagus and stomach.

Coffee: A link between coffee drinking and cancer of the bladder, pancreas, esophagus, and kidney has been suggested, but a causal effect is far from established.

Maximum tolerable limits have been established for contaminants.

Carcinogens cause cancer; mutagens initiate genetic changes. Because animal testing of carcinogens is time and money consuming, mutagen studies in bacteria assume the mechanism is the same as in human cancer. Flavonoids found in some food plants and in tea, coffee, cocoa, beer, and red wine are mutagens.

Summary of additives and contaminants:

- Saccharin.
- Cyclamates.
- BHT (butylated hydroxytoluene) and BHA (butylated hydroxyanisole) are antioxidants and preservatives. In lab tests, BHT may have a limited tumor-promoting effect.
- Vinylchloride used in packaging is associated with human cancers in individuals with high occupational exposure.
- DES (diethylstilbestrol), an estrogenic hormone, was used as a growth

promoter for cattle and sheep. It was used in pregnant women to prevent miscarriage, but induced vaginal cancer in their female children.

- Pesticides including DDT, Dieldrin, Lindane, Chlordane, and parathion all produce cancer in various laboratory animals.
- PCBs (polychlorinated biphenyls), used for a variety of industrial purposes, are carcinogenic in laboratory rodents and may be related to malignant melanoma tumors in humans.
- PAHs (polycyclic aromatic hydrocarbons), such as benzo(a)pyrene found in smoked or grilled meats, may be related to stomach cancer.

Of the enormous number of environmental contaminants that find their way into food, few appear to provoke human cancer, but it is difficult to confirm low-level hazards of this type.

Inhibitors of Carcinogens

In laboratory experiments, the common food additive BHA blocks tumor induction by known carcinogens. Chemically BHA is a phenol.

Indole-3-acetonitrile and aromatic isothiocyanates, found in brussels sprouts, cabbage, cauliflower, and broccoli (cruciferous vegetables), inhibit cancer formation in mice exposed to cancer producing agents.

Flavones found in fruits and vegetables; protease inhibitors found in many plants, seeds, soybeans, and lima beans; and betasitosterol, found in vegetable oils, are all protective.

How they act is unclear. Biochemically they must prevent the gene damage that causes in turn abnormal cell and tumor production. Results in animal or bacterial studies cannot be fully equated with human biology.

The Epidemiology of Cancer—The Study of Patterns of Disease

Ninety percent of human cancers appear to be environmental in origin, diet accounting for 60 percent of cancers in women and 40

116

percent in men. Diet affects tumor potential in the gastrointestinal tract (esophagus, stomach, small and large intestines, liver, and pancreas), male and female reproductive organs (breast, uterus, and prostate gland), bladder, and lungs.

Geography

Numerous observations have been made about the changing incidence of cancer in migrant groups. One of the classic examples is the decrease in cancer of the stomach and the increase in cancer of the colon and breast in Japanese who migrate to the United States, compared to those who remain in Japan. Similar studies have been done on Eastern Europeans coming to North America, Icelanders to Canada, and Southern Europeans to Australia. The change in cancer rates parallels the assimilation of the immigrant group into the social patterns and diet of the new country. Geography, that is, environment, far more than ethnic or genetic factors, is the major determinant of cancer.

Factors Affecting Cancer Rate

Several factors have produced an apparent increase in the cancer rate over the last quarter century. Improved diagnosis and improved record collecting and reporting may produce a false impression of an increased rate. The total number of cases rises as the total size of the population increases. There is an increase in the number of cases in proportion to the increasing age of the population, the elderly people who earlier in the century might have succumbed to infectious disease or cardiovascular disease before reaching the high cancer decades. Corrected for the changing age of the population, the true cancer rate for most organs appears remarkably unchanged in the last quarter century despite the increased complexity and presumed hostility of our chemical environment. The exception is the great increase in lung cancer, attributed to cigarette smoking. Stomach cancer has dropped substantially during the last quarter to half century, possibly related to changes in food preservation techniques and methods of preparation. Cervical cancer has shown a substantial drop in incidence and mortality, as a result of the early detection of precancerous lesions by the Pap smear. Most other cancers show little longterm change in incidence.

Cancer and
Socioeconomic Status

Colon and rectal cancer, postmenopausal breast cancer, and kidney cancer seem to correlate with higher socioeconomic status, which may in turn be a function of diet.

Cancer and
Religious Groups

Seventh Day Adventists, who follow a diet of milk, eggs, and vegetables and abstain from smoking and drinking have less colon cancer and to some extent less breast cancer. Mormons who follow similar practices and also consume modest amounts of meat have fewer stomach, colon, and female reproductive organ cancers.

A correlation between diet and cancer has been reported by many medical sources. The recurring pattern is that less meat and fat intake is associated with less cancer of the colon and rectum and of the reproductive organs. The hormone content of animal fat may be the relevant factor in causing reproductive organ cancer.

A long list of correlations between dietary patterns and specific cancers can be amassed: high animal fat diet and colon, rectum, breast, uterus, ovary, and prostate cancer; alcohol consumption and mouth and larynx cancer; beer consumption and rectal cancer.

Cancer—
Organ by Organ

Up to now we have been looking at possible causes of cancer in the different organs any given substance might affect. It is interesting to turn the data around and look at the various possible cancer causes by organ.

Esophageal cancer: Alcohol, tobacco, pickled food, food contaminated with molds containing mycotoxins or N-nitroso compounds. Diets high in fruits and vegetables appear to be protective.

Stomach cancer: High in Japan, associated with pickled foods. High in areas containing nitrates in drinking water. High in Iceland in association with the consumption of smoked foods. Protection may be afforded by green and yellow vegetables, milk, and foods containing Vitamin C.

118

Colon and rectal cancer: Many studies implicate total fat or animal (saturated) fat. There appears to be a protective effect from dietary fiber and cruciferous vegetables.

Liver cancer: Liver cancer appears to be related to intake of foods contaminated with aflatoxin; alcoholic cirrhosis of the liver; and is secondary to chronic hepatitis B infection.

Pancreatic cancer: Meat consumption, alcohol, and coffee have been implicated but without substantial statistical evidence.

Lung cancer: Cigarette smoking is, of course, the accepted primary cause of lung cancer but patterns of food consumption also play a role. There appears to be a significant protective effect from foods containing Vitamin A and its precursor, beta-carotene. Studies are not available evaluating the effect of pure Vitamin A, or beta-carotene, so again we caution that the truly protective substance may be some other, unidentified factor in those foods other than Vitamin A itself.

Urinary bladder cancer: Saccharin use and coffee have been associated with bladder cancer but a definite cause or relationship in humans has not been established.

Breast cancer: A large number of factors are associated with breast cancer. Diet plays an important role. A high-fat diet is associated with increased risk of breast cancer.

Cancer of the uterus: Cancer of the uterus correlates with increased fat in the diet and closely parallels cancers of the breast, ovary, colon, and rectum in that respect. A transient increase in uterine cancer during the 1970s was related to the use of estrogens during menopause.

Ovarian cancer is related to high-fat diets.

Prostate cancer is also related to high-fat diets.

Doll and Peto in 1981 collected a number of estimates from the medical literature varying from 10 to 70 percent of cancers that could be reduced by dietary changes. Their own estimate was 35 percent reduction of deaths from cancer by purely dietary modifications.

Cancer Organ	Percent of Decrease Possible by Diet
Stomach	90
Large bowel	90

Cancer

Organ	Percent of Decrease Possible by Diet
Uterus	50
Gallbladder	50
Pancreas	50
Breast	50
Lung	20
Larynx	20
Bladder	20
Cervix	20
Mouth	20
Esophagus	20
All other sites	10

The dietary changes called for are neither extreme nor impractical. It's worth it!

TWENTY

THE CAUSES OF CANCER: AVOIDABLE RISKS IN YOUR LIFESTYLE

Cancer is an avoidable disease arising from lifestyle, environment, and diet.

U.S. Cancer Deaths 1978	Organ
400,000	Total
95,000	Lung
53,000	Colon and rectum
35,000	Breast cancer
22,000	Prostate
21,000	Pancreas
14,000	Stomach

Together the six leading cancers accounted for 60 percent of all cancer deaths, with the remaining 40 percent accounted for by 30 other types of tumors. Avoidable causes of cancer include naturally occurring and manmade carcinogens, viruses, excesses or deficiencies in diet, sexual activities (cervical cancer associated with genital herpes and Kaposi's sarcoma associated with acquired immune deficiency syndrome), and a number of other factors. Direct study of human populations has provided provocative clues about the origin of cancer. Studies of large groups of people who moved from one country to another and experienced marked changes in their susceptibility to different cancers have suggested cause and effect relationships, especially in the important area of dietary changes. Another useful technique is to study areas that are particularly high or low in a given type of cancer and try to identify some aspect of lifestyle as a causative or preventive factor. For example, why is esophageal cancer high in Iran and low in Nigeria, or stomach cancer high in Japan and low in Uganda? What explains the high rate of prostate cancer in United States blacks and the low rate in Japanese? Breast cancer is high in British Columbia, Canada, and low in the non-Jewish population in Israel. Colon cancer is high in Connecticut and low in Nigeria, bladder cancer high in Connecticut and low in Japan. For uterine cancer the rate is high in California and low in Japan. Japanese and whites in Hawaii have similar esophageal and stomach cancer rates, far less than the rates in Japan. For colon, rectum, prostate, and breast, the rates in Japan are far lower. Cervical cancer is higher in Japan, uterine cancer and ovarian cancer lower. For lung cancer, Japanese in Hawaii have a higher rate than in Japan but not nearly as high as white residents of Hawaii, possibly due to the time lag between adopting white smoking habits and the development of lung cancer.

Data collection and interpretation is often difficult. Accuracy of diagnosis and completeness of reporting are not uniform around the country or around the world. Increasing age of the population must also be corrected for. Improvements in treatment may affect the death rate, although not the incidence of certain cancers.

Provocative changes in the occurrence of different cancers around the world have occurred during the last 25 years; for example, the increase in esophageal cancer in blacks living in South Africa; the epidemic increase in lung cancer associated with smoking; the occurrence of mesothelioma, a cancer of the lungs and pleura associated with asbestos; the decrease in tongue cancer in England; and the decrease in cancer of the cervix and stomach in Western Europe and North America.

Scientific proof of cause and effect is difficult because of the obvious complexities of doing controlled, valid statistical studies in large numbers of people subjected to a variety of lifestyle factors. Evidence is most often circumstantial, for example, the drop in the rate of cancer of the bladder in chemical workers since 2-

naphthylamine production was stopped; or the lung cancer risk in cigarette smokers that becomes similar to that of nonsmokers after cigarette smoking is stopped.

Increased cancer rates are seen with increasing age. Genetic factors may also play a role. For example, skin cancer is more common in whites than in blacks. People who have Type A blood group have 20 percent more cancer of the stomach than persons with Type O. Orientals have less leukemia but more cancers of the nose and throat.

The most common cancer in the United States, lung cancer, has more than doubled in the last quarter century because of cigarette smoking. Breast, colon, and rectum cancers vary from country to country, correlating strikingly with fat consumption.

Other established causes of cancer:

Agent	Organ
aflatoxin	liver
alcohol	head and neck
	esophagus
	liver
asbestos	lung
	pleura
radiation	bone marrow
estrogen	uterus
obesity	uterus
	gallbladder
phenacetin	kidney
late age of first pregnancy	breast
low number of pregnancies	ovary
parasites (certain)	bladder
	liver
large number of sexual partners	cervix
tobacco	head and neck
	lung
	esophagus
	bladder
vinyl chloride	liver
Hepatitis B virus	liver

Recapitulation—
Avoidable Causes
of Cancer

Tobacco

Tobacco causes one third of the deaths among males from cancer of the mouth, larynx, esophagus, and bladder and 90 percent of male deaths from lung cancer. Male cigar and pipe smokers have a risk similar to cigarette smokers for mouth cancer. There are an estimated 54 million cigarette smokers in the United States. Professionals and business executives are less likely to smoke or, if they do smoke, are more likely to use filtered cigarettes, or only cigars or pipes. Public health efforts need to be directed at low-income groups, teenagers, and young women, as well as middle-class males. Following cessation of smoking, the risk of cancer of the mouth and larynx, esophagus, lung, and bladder decreases steadily and, after 10 to 15 years, is about the same as for lifelong nonsmokers.

Cancer risk, particularly for lung cancer, increases in proportion to the number of cigarettes smoked per day, with even 1 to 10 cigarettes producing a marked increase in risk compared to that of nonsmokers. Cancer risk also increases with the length of time the individual has smoked.

Smoking cessation programs involve a variety of individual or group techniques. Longterm cessation success is variable, with one-year success rates of up to 44 percent in established heavy smokers. Campaigns focused on not starting smoking in teenagers have had success rates of 67 percent. Decreasing the carcinogenity of a cigarette by using filters, decreasing the amount of tar and nicotine, and not smoking the cigarette down to a short stub are improvements, providing the number of cigarettes smoked does not increase proportionately with the decrease in nicotine per cigarette.

Death rates from lung cancer in women continue to climb, from 4.6 per 100,000 in 1950 to 20.9 per 100,000 in 1982. For 1983, lung cancer deaths in women numbered 34,000 (17 percent of all female cancer deaths), second only to breast cancer deaths: 37,000 (18 percent).

In 1982, there were 129,000 tobacco-related cancer deaths, about one third of all cancer deaths.

In 1959, 53 percent of American adults smoked cigarettes.

124

Thirty-three percent still do, but for physicians the figure has dropped from 53 to 10 percent, striking evidence of the importance doctors attach to nonsmoking.

Alcohol

Heavy alcohol consumption is associated with cancer of the mouth, pharynx, esophagus, and liver. Alcohol and tobacco appear to have a synergistic effect, together having a higher cancer incidence than either alone. Heavy drinking is defined as 1.6 or more ounces of alcohol per day, the equivalent of 4 ounces of whiskey, 16 ounces of wine or 32 ounces of beer. Heavy smoking is defined for the purpose of this analysis as over 40 cigarettes, 20 pipefuls of tobacco, or 5 cigars per day.

Food

Breast cancer: Mortality rates are six times greater in North Americans than in some Asian and African peoples. Fat in the diet appears to be the crucial variable. Japanese women and vegetarian women in the United States who eat less animal fat and meat have much less breast cancer.

Colon cancer: Connecticut men have a one in thirty chance of developing cancer of the colon by age 74. In Colombia, South America, and Nigeria, Africa, the risks are 1 in 300 and 1 in 700. Japanese in Hawaii, once they adopt western patterns of diet, assume the higher colon cancer rates of the local population.

Colon cancer rates are closely associated with the amounts of beef and dietary fat consumed. The highest rates in the world for colon cancer are seen in Argentina, Uruguay, and New Zealand, countries known for their beef consumption. Seventh Day Adventists in the United States who eat no meat have the lowest rates.

Dietary fiber, the remnants of the plant cell wall remaining after digestion, and present in larger quantities than crude fiber, increases stool bulk. Diets high in fiber appear to protect against colon cancer by diluting carcinogens in the stool and by provoking rapid transit time and excretion. In rural areas of Finland unrefined grain products are a staple, and the incidence of colon and rectal cancer is low. In Copenhagen cereal consumption consists largely of refined grains, and the incidence of colon and rectum cancer is high. Diets high in fat stimulate gallbladder production of bile acids, from which intestinal bacteria form carcinogens. Higher colon cancer rates parallel the amount of dihydroxycholanic acid produced by colon bacteria.

Stomach cancer: Cancer of the stomach and cancer of the colon seem to have an inverse relationship. Colon cancer is often associated with affluent cultures consuming large amounts of beef and fat, whereas stomach cancer is more prevalent in less affluent regions, where the diets are higher in starch. Japan, Iceland, Chile, and Finland have high stomach cancer rates. New Zealand, Australia, and the United States have low rates. Migrating populations change their stomach cancer rates to that of the new country within one generation. In the United States the rate 50 years ago was 30 males and 22 females per 100,000 population. The current rate is 7.5 males and 3.7 females.

The Japanese stomach cancer rate appears to be related to their consumption of pickled vegetables and dried, salted fish. The incidence of stomach cancer dropped substantially among Japanese who changed to a fresh vegetable and fruit diet.

Vitamins in food: Vitamins C and E, by their antioxidant effect, inhibit the formation of *N*-nitroso compounds, potent gastric carcinogens. Vitamin A (retinol), synthetic retinoids, and carotenoids are important in the normal reproduction and development of the cells lining the gastrointestinal, urinary, reproductive, and respiratory systems. A study in Norway in which a large number of men were followed for five years showed that those with high Vitamin A intake had 60 to 80 percent fewer lung cancers than those with low Vitamin A consumption. In a similar study in Japan 280,000 persons were followed for 10 years. Those smokers who had a high daily consumption of yellow and green vegetables, which are high in retinoids, had 20 to 30 percent fewer lung cancers. In high dosage, natural retinoids are toxic to the liver and blood levels are limited by saturation of retinol binding protein, the transport mechanism for Vitamin A in the bloodstream. Its stable concentration acts as a governor on blood Vitamin A levels. There are efforts to synthesize retinoids to bypass the problems.

Body Chemistry

To produce cell damage, many cancer causing agents must become metabolically active—the chemical process of oxidation—

producing what are known as free radicals and excited molecular oxygen. Substances that interfere with the process include selenium, Vitamin E, and beta-carotene.

Selenium levels have been found to be low in some cancer patients. Selenium is toxic if taken in excessive amounts, so indiscriminate consumption is not recommended. Vitamin E is found naturally occurring in so many foods that true low Vitamin E states are uncommon. Studies of people who regularly consume large amounts of Vitamin E have not shown a distinct protective effect against cancer.

Each molecule of beta-carotene (provitamin A) is convertible in the body into two molecules of Vitamin A. At least twenty dietary studies show a protective effect against cancer of diets high in foods containing beta-carotene.

Is the beta-carotene protective, or is there some unidentified constituent in foods high in beta-carotene that is actually the protective agent? Or do people who consume high vegetable diets as a result consume fewer meats and animal fats, the cancer-provocative foods?

In cell cultures and experimental animals, Vitamin A (retinol) and related substances (retinoids), inhibit initiated cell cancers from being promoted into clinical cancers. In humans, except in rare Vitamin A deficiency states, taking Vitamin A even in large quantities approaching toxicity does not change the blood level of circulating Vitamin A. Estrogens are one of the few substances that appear to affect Vitamin A levels, and women who take estrogen itself or with progesterone in oral contraceptives have higher Vitamin A levels in the blood. Although there is some evidence of less ovarian and uterine cancer (and no increase in breast cancer) in women who have taken birth control pills, menopausal and postmenopausal use of estrogens increases the risk of breast and uterine cancer.

Overnutrition: In mice undernutrition corresponds with less cancer and longer lifespan. In humans overnutrition and obesity correlate with an increased death risk from some cancers.

Cancer of the uterus (the endometrium) is strongly related to overnutrition, a result of hormone conversion (adrenal to female or estrogenic) in fatty tissue, the major source of estrogens in postmenopausal women.

Breast cancer is related to fat intake, colon and rectal cancer to fat and meat intake—observations made in studies around the world.

In males, obesity is a risk factor for prostate cancer. The mechanism of action is not clear despite epidemiologic study in humans or laboratory study in animals and cell cultures.

Food Additives

Chemicals added to food as preservatives or to affect color, flavor, and so on, involve enormous numbers of substances. Three common ones are particularly important: saccharin causes bladder cancer in rats; BHT (butylated hydroxytoluene), an antioxidant, increases lung tumors caused by urethane in mice but inhibits some carcinogens in cell studies; nitrites, meat preservatives, when converted to nitrosamines in the stomach, may cause stomach cancer.

For these food additives, evidence of cancer provocation in humans is indirect, but prudence dictates their avoidance.

Sexual and Reproductive
Effects on Cancer

A woman's risk of developing cancer of the cervix, the number of her sexual partners, and her chance of having a herpes virus infection appear related.

Pregnancy and childbirth have a beneficial effect. Women who have had children early in their lives have less cancer of the breast, ovary, and uterus.

Occupation

Since the susceptibility of chimney sweeps to scrotal cancer was first described in 1775, many other occupational causes of cancer have been identified:

- Bladder cancer in dye, rubber, and coal gas workers, from contact with aromatic amines.
- Skin and lung cancer in metallurgy workers, from arsenic.
- Lung and pleural cancer in asbestos workers.
- Prostate cancer in cadmium workers.
- Bone marrow cancer in radiologists.
- Skin, scrotum, and lung cancer from exposure to petroleum derivatives, such as tar and asphalt, containing polycyclic hydrocarbons.
- Liver cancer in PVC manufacturers using vinyl chloride.

128

Of the 400,000 cancer deaths in the United States in 1978, about 17,000 have been attributed to occupational causes.

Pollution

Air, water, and food pollution means substances generated by man:

- Products of (hydrocarbon fuel) combustion pumped into the air from car exhausts and factory smokestacks.
- Mercury compounds discharged into the sea from factories and consumed by shellfish, then eaten by humans.
- Pesticides used for agricultural purposes, which then enter the food cycle.

Hard evidence about direct cause and effect relationships between pollutants and human cancer is hard to come by. Theoretically they play a role in individual cases of high exposure. They may also act in concert with each other, although each is low in concentration, and may act as promoters of tumors initiated by other mechanisms.

Industrial products with which the average person has daily contact are often derivatives of the petroleum and chemical industries, including cosmetics and hair dyes, plastic products, organic solvents, cleaning fluids, paints, and ink. The possibility that some of the hundreds or thousands of products may not be biologically inert is a real one, but very few data exist. That such products possess carcinogenic potential enough to induce cancer is possible, but is difficult to prove. On balance the majority of agents are probably not clinically hazardous.

Medicines

A number of drugs and medical procedures are known to cause human cancer, including radiation, estrogen, phenacetin, ultraviolet light, and some drugs and radiation therapy used in the treatment of cancer itself.

Estimates place the number of deaths from diagnostic radiation at between 2,000 and 4,500 of the 400,000 U.S. cancer deaths per year, an amount equal to about one percent of all cancer deaths. The number should decrease as physicians and patients become more aware of the risk.

The large increase in the incidence of endometrial (uterine) cancer during the mid-1970s has been attributed to the use of estrogens for the relief of menopausal and postmenopausal symptoms. Uterine cancer accounts for one percent of all cancer deaths and the proportion of those due to estrogen use is probably less than half. Physician and patient awareness has diminished use of estrogen for this purpose.

The birth control pill may decrease the risk of ovarian cancer. There is no conclusive evidence of an increase in breast or cervical cancer rates.

Sunlight and
Natural Radiation

Sunlight causes various skin cancers, including basal cell carcinoma and squamous cell carcinoma, neither of which is serious, and melanoma, a very malignant tumor.

Naturally existing background ionizing radiation has been estimated to result in 5,500 cancer deaths per year, about 1.4 percent of the total. With the exception of melanoma deaths due to sun bathing, deaths from sunlight or natural radiation are unavoidable.

Viral Agents

Because of the resemblance of viral particles to the genetic apparatus of human cells, a link between viruses and cancer is being sought. When viral DNA enters a human cell it affects the reproduction of the cell. Cervical cancer may be an example, and liver cancer may result after Hepatitis B virus infection.

Other Factors

Stress, breakdown of immune mechanisms, and exercise are being studied. A definite relationship has not been proven. In the case of stress, while unproven, chronic socioeconomic deprivation may in males lead to suppression of immune system function, which in turn allows tumor development.

Summary

The proportion of cancer deaths from various identified causes is as follows:

Cause	Percent
Tobacco	30 (some estimates up to 40%)
Alcohol	3
Diet	35 (some estimates up to 70%)

Those three factors alone account for 2 of 3 cancer deaths, or 267,000 of the 400,000 Americans who will die this year from cancer. The knowledge to produce a dramatic decrease in the death toll from cancer in the 1980s and 1990s is available. When added to the decreased death rate from cardiovascular disease of the 1970s, the impact of changes in lifestyle on health and longevity is incredible.

For other agents involved in cancer initiation or promotion, the percentages of total cancer deaths break down as follows:

Cause	Percent
Food additives	Less than 1
Reproductive and sexual activity	7
Occupation	4
Pollution	2
Industrial products	Less than 1
Medicines and medical procedures	1
Radiation & ultraviolet exposure	3
Infection and unknown causes	Up to 10

Influencing Lifestyle

Tobacco and alcohol use, food habits, occupation, and lifestyle affect our chances of getting cancer. When physicians, public health agencies, and the media campaign in concert, individuals do make changes in their lifestyles. The extraordinary decrease of 25 percent in the mortality rate from cardiovascular disease over the last decade is evidence that the public will take notice of public health messages. Outstanding medical authorities agree that it is changes in lifestyle—losing weight, decreasing the amount of fat in the diet, exercise, cessation of cigarette smoking, and acceptance of blood pressure treatment—that is saving lives, far more than are emergency rooms and intensive care units, coronary artery bypass surgery, and new medicines.

The need to get the message out about cancer should now be number one in urgency.

131

TWENTY-ONE

DOES BETA-CAROTENE PREVENT CANCER?

Great care must be taken in interpreting data. In a number of studies it was found that a high blood retinol (Vitamin A) level or consumption of beta-carotene foods correlates with a below average risk of cancer. There are possible flaws in jumping from epidemiology (observations about large human populations) to the conclusion that consuming large amounts of beta-carotene-containing foods or Vitamin A capsules in an effort to raise the retinol blood level will have a beneficial effect. Changes in retinol levels may simply reflect a secondary reaction, with another factor responsible for the change in cancer risk. Or people who like to eat vegetables may eat less of carcinogenic foods, particularly meat and fat. There are, however, well over 300 research papers confirming the impact of retinoids and carotenoids on cancer:

- In the laboratory on the behavior of cancerous cell cultures (induced by viruses, chemicals, and radiation).
- In preventing or delaying cancer in animals that have been exposed to carcinogens.
- In antagonizing the malignant effects of tumor promoters in cell culture and animal experiments.
- In causing the regression of precancerous lesions in man.

The impact of retinoids and carotenoids seems to be on the tumor *promotion* phase in the development of cancer, a crucial point, because the *initiation* phase of a cancer may be followed by a latent period of decades before promotion occurs with the development of a full-fledged clinical cancer. Retinoids may have valuable human application, even at a late point in the cancer process.

In addition to epidemiologic or retrospective observations and cell culture and animal experiments, the best scientific evidence would come from well controlled, future human studies. But comparing large, randomly selected equivalent groups of people, varying only in their diet or consumption of retinoid or carotenoid capsules, is difficult. The cost and time factors of such studies are high. A study using American physicians as subjects recently got underway, but any results will not be available for years.

Serum studies in India, Pakistan, East Africa, Britain, and the United States showed that cancer patients had lower blood retinol levels than control patients. Beta-carotene levels were also measured in several studies and were also found to be lower in cancer patients than in the controls.

A study in Japan of 265,118 Japanese began in 1965. All completed detailed dietary questionnaires. By 1975, 807 had died of lung cancer. The risk of dying from lung cancer was 40% less for those who ate vegetables containing beta-carotene daily than for those who ate them less often. Daily use of the vegetables was also associated with a lower rate of stomach and prostate cancer. The consumption of yellow and green vegetables amounted to more than half of the beta-carotene in the diet of the subjects studied.

Questionnaires about smoking and diet were completed by 8,278 Norwegian men during the middle sixties; this group was monitored for five years. Low consumption of beta-carotene-containing foods was predictive of higher lung cancer rates. In a similar study involving 40,000 people in Norway and Minnesota, beginning in the middle to late sixties, preliminary results are promising. In a Chicago group of 2,000 people who completed a diet diary in 1959, a 19-year follow-up showed a lower cancer risk associated with higher beta-carotene intake (preliminary analysis).

A lower cancer risk, although not statistically significant, was reported in medical journals in 1978 and 1980 for people using Vitamin A pills. Roswell Park Memorial Institute in Buffalo, New York, studied thousands of cancer patients and controls. The risk of lung, bladder, esophageal, and laryngeal cancer increased as the beta-carotene-containing foods decreased. Other studies have been inconclusive, contradictory, or inadequately controlled. In some reports the specific pattern of foods consumed was lacking, as were estimates of beta-carotene or retinol intake.

In a study on esophageal cancer in Iran, the tumor was frequent in areas where vegetables and fruits were notably lacking in the diet. Studies on stomach, colon, and rectal cancers in Norway and the United States showed higher cancer rates where vegetable intake was low. In Liverpool, England, increased gastrointestinal cancer occurred when green vegetables were consumed less than weekly.

Many studies of beta-carotene diets and cancer in humans are flawed, lacking large numbers of patients, sufficient duration of follow-up, accurate reporting of diet intake, and so on. Most are retrospective, looking back over a number of years at whatever diet and cancer data could be identified. Such studies are not the result of faulty research but an attempt to save time, to extract information from existing data often collected with other purposes in mind. Valid future studies have the disadvantage that conclusions must wait many years. Before turning our backs on hindsight, heed the words of Peto and Doll, et al., "The perfect may well be the enemy of the relevant." If we disregard information because of its imperfections, we may be overlooking for a decade a crucial breakthrough in cancer prevention and treatment. The laboratory worker must go hand in hand with the epidemiologist. Each should suggest new avenues of research and verification to the other. Each plays a role: cell cultures and animal experiments, retrospective (epidemiology) and prospective (statistically planned) studies. Each may spin off insights on the chemistry of cancer or clinical information on carotenoid/retinoid prevention of cancer.

We know that beta-carotene "quenches the excitation energy of singlet oxygen and traps certain organic free radicals" (Peto and Doll, et al.). Its anticancer effect may reside in the deactivation of chemical reactions, preventing the oxidative damage they cause. In deciphering the beta-carotene mechanism we may be unveiling the mechanism of cancer, the biochemical and genetic aberration within the human cell.

In Brazil and West Africa, some parts of the population consume large quantities of red palm oil, an oil extremely high in beta-carotene. Studies relating beta-carotene intake, blood level, and relationship to cancer are in progress in Brazil. We expect an association between low vegetable use and high cancer risk. We expect an inverse relationship between serum beta-carotene and retinol, and cancer. The issues are how much benefit, and clarification of cause and effect. High daily doses of Vitamin A, 25,000 to 50,000 per day, produce toxicity in a matter of months. The recommended daily intake of Vitamin A is 5,000 IU. Beta-carotene in doses we now consider high is not toxic. Most people ingest only a few milligrams a day of beta-carotene, but up to 200 milligrams per day are used in the treatment of a rare disorder known as erythropoietic protoporphyria, without ill effect. West Africans and Brazilians who use red palm oil in cooking have very high levels of liver retinol and blood carotene, but their blood retinol is normal because of the blood retinol regulating mechanism. Retinol binding protein functions as a transport mechanism for Vitamin A (retinol) and when fully saturated can and will accept no more, acting as a control mechanism for blood Vitamin A levels.

Consumption of Vitamin A or its precursor, beta-carotene, or foods containing them does not significantly change blood Vitamin A levels. Individuals with high blood retinol have less cancer; those with low retinol have more cancer. High beta-carotene in the diet correlates with high beta-carotene blood levels and less cancer. That may be because of beta-carotene itself or retinol, or to some other substance that exists in the same foods as beta-carotene. It may be that people eating large quantities of vegetables containing beta-carotene eat less meat and animal fats, which lowers cancer risk.

In addition to cell research, animal studies, and retrospective data, we need large-scale prospective studies of beta-carotene and retinol in food and capsule form, and correlation with blood levels and cancer rates in subjects and controls over a 5 to 10 year period.

Fortunately the beta-carotene effect appears to be on the promotion stage of cancer genesis rather than on the initiation stage. Because initiation may be followed by a latency period measured in decades, any effects on initiation will help only the very young and future generations. Examination of retrospective data shows cancer rates can change within a few years; therefore, beta-carotene must interfere with the promotion phase of the cancer process. Individuals of any age may benefit.

Why not just take beta-carotene or Vitamin A in capsule form? What amount shall we take? Are there toxic levels for beta-carotene, as we know there are for Vitamin A? Will beta-carotene synthetically produced or processed from foods be identical to that found naturally in foods? By analogy total cholesterol was considered to be the key substance in evaluating coronary artery disease risk. Now a fraction of the total cholesterol known as HDL (high density lipoprotein) is regarded as vital in the coronary artery risk profile. Soon an HDL fraction (apolipoproteins) may displace HDL as the key to the blood fat and coronary disease issue.

Are there catalysts, substances that activate or enhance the actions of beta-carotene, found in association with it in foods, substances that have not yet been identified? In purified form without such a catalyst present, the beta-carotene effect might be ineffective or blocked. Is beta-carotene actually the key substance in the foods in which it is found? Perhaps it is just the vehicle that transports in chemical combination another yet unidentified substance, the actual active ingredient. Perhaps another substance occurs in the same distribution of foods as beta-carotene, a substance that actually is the one affecting cancer risk, and beta-carotene itself is just coincidentally present. Does beta-carotene have its effect because large consumption of beta-carotene foods is associated with less consumption of meats and animal fats, which decreases cancer risk? Another issue in taking beta-carotene supplements, even if effective against cancer, is that an unstructured diet may be inadequate from other nutritional and health standpoints. Our information about an anticancer effect is derived from observation of dietary practices, not from monitoring chemical supplements. If we are to act on the emerging beta-carotene dietary concept now, it would be best to mimic the epidemiologic routes observed, not to take an uncharted biochemical detour.

Should we wait for ultimate proof of the beta-carotene effect on lowering the risk of cancer? Cardiovascular disease is an outstanding guideline. In the last decade the death rate from cardiovascular disease dropped by 25 percent. Two million Americans die each year, of them one million from cardiovascular disease. Had the cardiovascular death rate of the 1950s and 1960s continued during the 1970s, one and a quarter million Americans would have died from heart disease in 1980 instead of the one million who did, a saving of one quarter of a million lives per year.

How did that come about? In the 1970s, in response to physicians, public health agencies, and the public information media, books, magazines, newspapers, radio and television, the American public was made aware that changes in lifestyle appeared to be beneficial. The changes included exercise, weight loss, limiting animal fat in the diet, cessation of cigarette smoking, and more aggressive treatment of high blood pressure. Absolute proof was lacking, particularly about the advice to limit animal fats and cholesterol in the diet, but large numbers of people complied, to their benefit.

An adequate study of dietary changes and cardiovascular disease may be close to impossible from a practical standpoint. It would require a large number of patients divided into a test group and a control group, followed for many years by a large number of physicians. A large number of variables, both known and unsuspected, would be involved. Studies requiring control of diets in human beings obviously cannot be regulated with the same degree of confidence as controlling the food intake of a laboratory animal. Such studies will always fall short of meeting a statistician's concept of perfection. What is called for is an informed judgment that a high degree of probability of benefit exists, and that careful examination does not suggest any harm in the intended approach. In the case of cardiovascular disease these criteria were met and a decade of time and a quarter of a million lives a year were salvaged, a form of proof which might never have been achieved had a conventional, prospective study approach been elected. The prospective study is a valuable tool and one that should not be bypassed in the great majority of research endeavors. Where possible it should be attempted simultaneously with the approach used for cardiovascular disease, plus cellular biology studies, animal research, and retrospective epidemiology. Cancer and cardiovascular disease have certain similarities from a research standpoint. Because of urgency and because diet is the central issue, I propose a mass effort similar to that for cardiovascular disease in the 1970s be undertaken in the 1980s for cancer. While other research methods proceed, in the next five to ten years we can save millions of lives. The probable benefits are high and the risks appear low.

We have many precedents in medical history for such actions. William Withering treated heart failure with foxglove, a plant growing in the garden of an old woman in Shropshire, England, long before pharmacologic science could extract and identify digitalis, its active ingredient. Ignaz Semmelweis in the General Hospital of

Vienna saved the lives of thousands of women dying in childbirth by insisting on handwashing by doctors before deliveries. He recognized that obstetricians themselves were introducing something lethal from their hands into the bodies of women in labor, long before the science of bacteriology identified the germs causing childbed fever. Immunization against smallpox, pasteurization of milk, and treatment of rabies all saved lives before their exact mechanisms were known.

Mankind is lucky—we get a second chance when it comes to cardiovascular disease. Even prolonged cigarette smoking, obesity, high-cholesterol diets, and untreated high blood pressure will not produce irreversible cardiovascular disease for many decades. With even belated treatment and reversal of risk factors, we may live on in cardiovascular health. For cancer it appears much the same. The fault lies not within ourselves in genetic flaws but, as is heart disease, cancer is imposed on us from outside. But with knowledge we can take steps to protect our genetic strength and reach for the health and longevity that evolution has written into our chromosomes.

Happily, prevention of cancer and heart disease are not at odds, another gift of evolution. The same risk factors, diet and cigarette smoking, apply to both. The antidisease diet is perhaps not unlike that of our primitive forebears. We can only begin to guess at the possible lifespan of man, with infection controlled by antibiotics, immunizations, pure food and water, and good sanitation. With heart disease and cancer about to be mastered, these last decades of the twentieth century will be remembered less for technological and industrial progress but more for our changing lifestyle.

BIBLIOGRAPHY

"The Active Herb Could Be No Other Than the Foxglove." *Journal of Cardiovascular Medicine*, February 1982, pp. 164–65.

Atkins, R.C., M.D., *Dr. Atkins' Diet Revolution*, New York: Bantam Books, 1981.

Berenblum, Isaac, M.D., "The Mechanism of Carcinogenesis: A Study of the Significance of Cocarcinogenic Action and Related Phenomena." *Cancer Research 1*, 1941, pp. 807–14.

Berland, T., "Debunking Those Dieting Myths." *Better Homes and Gardens*, July 1982, pp. 17–20.

Berland, T., and the editors of *Consumer Guide*, "Rating the Diets." New York: Signet Books, 1979.

Berwick, D., M.D., "The Evidence Against Cholesterol." *Journal of Cardiovascular Medicine*, February 1981, pp. 151–53.

Borhani, N.O., M.D., "The Case for Diet Modification to Retard Atherosclerosis." *Journal of Cardiovascular Medicine*, December 1980, pp. 1085–89.

Brauer, A., "Dr. Denis P. Burkitt, The Apostle of Fiber." *MD*, January 1983, pp. 107–15.

Ca-A Cancer Journal for Clinicians, New York: American Cancer Society, Vols. 30–33, 1980–83.

The Cancer Institute Bulletin, Tufts Health Sciences Schools, New England Medical Center, Vol. 3, No. 1, Spring 1983.

Cancer Related Checkups, brochure and letter to the medical profession, American Cancer Society, 1980.

"Cigarette Smoking." editorial, *Medical Tribune,* June 29, 1983.

Coronary Risk Handbook, American Heart Association, 1973.

Crick, Francis and James D. Watson, letter published in *Nature,* April 25, 1953.

Diet and Coronary Disease, General Dietary Recommendations of the American Heart Association, Committee on Nutrition, 1973.

Diet, Nutrition, and Cancer, Committee on Diet, Nutrition, and Cancer, Assembly of Life Sciences, National Research Council, National Academy of Sciences, Washington, DC, 1982.

Dietary Goals for the United States, Select Committee on Nutrition and Human Needs, United States Senate, 1977.

"Does Life Style Cause Cancer?" symposium, *New York State Journal of Medicine,* July 1980, pp. 1237–58 and August 1980, pp. 1401–16.

Doll, R., and R. Peto, "The Causes of Cancer: Quantitative Estimates of Avoidable Risks of Cancer in the United States Today." *Journal of the National Cancer Institute,* Vol. 66, No. 6, June 1981, pp. 1192–1308.

Encyclopedia Americana, 1980, Vol. 1, "History of Agriculture," pp. 353–60; "Domestication of Animals," pp. 886–87.

Feinleib, M., M.D., et al., "The Changing Pattern of Ischemic Heart Disease." *The Journal of Cardiovascular Medicine,* Vol. 7, No. 2, February 1982, pp. 139–48.

Geographic Patterns in the Risk of Dying and Associated Factors Ages 35–74 Years, United States, 1968–72, Vital and Health Statistics, Series 3, No. 18, National Center for Health Statistics.

Gibbons, D.L., "The Worst Problem Is Pessimism," interview of V.T. DeVita, Jr., M.D., Director, National Cancer Institute, *Medical World News,* April 11, 1983, pp. 62–77.

The Good Food Guide. Better Homes and Gardens Creative Ideas, low calorie recipes, 1983, pp. 41–48.

Goodman, D.S., M.D., at the 1983 meeting of the American College of Physicians, Panel on Diet and Cardiovascular Disease, Comments against the necessity or practicality of absolute proof of the cholesterol-cardiovascular disease link, cited in *Internal Medicine News,* June 1–14, 1982, pp. 1 and 50.

Havas, S., M.D., and M.S. Honeyman, Ph.D., "Declines in Mortality in Connecticut 1960–1980." *Connecticut Health Bulletin,* Vol. 96, No. 2, 1982, pp. 152–58.

Hayflick, L., Ph.D., Comments on cell aging at the Duke University Center for the Study of Aging and Human Development, 25th Anniversary lecture series, cited by Mushak, B. in *Medical Tribune,* November 26, 1980, p. 10.

Highlights of the Surgeon General's Report on Smoking and Health. Morbidity and Mortality Weekly Report, Centers for Disease Control, Vol. 28, No. 1, January 12, 1979, pp. 1–12.

Jenkins, C.D., Ph.D., "Social Environment and Cancer Mortality in Men." *New England Journal of Medicine,* February 17, 1983.

Kannel, W.B., M.D., "Meaning of the Downward Trend in Cardiovascular Mortality." *Journal of the American Medical Association,* Vol. 247, No. 6, February 12, 1982, pp. 877–80, and editorial, p. 836.

Keys, A., et al., "Indices of Relative Weight and Obesity." *Journal of Chronic Diseases,* Vol. 25, 1972, pp. 329–43.

Kraus, B., *Calories and Carbohydrates,* New York: Signet Books, 1971.

Levy, R.I., M.D., "Cholesterol and Disease—What Are the Facts?" *The Journal of the American Medical Association* (editorial), Vol. 248, No. 21, December 3, 1982, pp. 2888–89.

Levy, R.I., M.D., "Cholesterol and Noncardiovascular Mortality." *The Journal of Cardiovascular Medicine,* NIH Reports, Vol. 5, No. 11, November 1980, pp. 960–64.

Lipsett, M.B., M.D., "Nutrition, Hormones, and Cancer." National Institutes of Health, *Medical Times,* Vol. 111, No. 5, May 1983, pp. 68–71.

Logan, J., and J. Cairns, "The Secrets of Cancer." *Nature*, Vol. 300, November 11, 1982, pp. 104–105.

"Lung Cancer in Women—Five Years Later, Situation Worse." (editorial), *New England Journal of Medicine*, August 18, 1983.

"Mammography: A Statement of the American Cancer Society." *Connecticut Medicine*, Vol. 47, No. 1, January 1983, pp. 37–39.

Mazel, J., *The Beverly Hills Diet*, New York: Berkley Books, 1981.

McKegney, F.P., M.D., "Psychoneuroimmunology: What Lies Ahead." *Drug Therapy*, August 1982, pp. 159–69.

Mirkin, G.B., M.D., and R.N. Shore, M.D., "The Beverly Hills Diet, Dangers of the Newest Weight Loss Fad." *Journal of the American Medical Association*, Vol. 246, No. 19, November 13, 1981, pp. 2235–37.

Nestle, M., Ph.D., "What Constitutes Good Nutrition, and for Whom." *Consultant*, January 1983, pp. 271–86.

"New Findings About Cancer Raising Hope." *The New York Times*, February 20, 1983, p. 1.

News and Views: "Anatomy of a Human Cancer Gene." *Nature*, Vol. 300, November 11, 1982, p. 103.

Nichols, W.S., M.D., and R.M. Nakamura, M.D., "The Latest Laboratory Tests for Cancer." *Consultant*, June 1981, pp. 131–39.

Nutrition and Your Health, Dietary Guidelines for Americans, U.S. Department of Agriculture and U.S. Department of Health, Education, and Welfare, February 1980.

Page, I.H., M.D., "Century of Changes, Challenges." cited in *The Internist*, November 1982, p. 7.

Pemberton, C.M., R.D., and C.F. Gastineau, M.D., Ph.D., eds., *Mayo Clinic Diet Manual*, 5th ed., Philadelphia: W.B. Saunders Co., 1981.

Peto, R., R. Doll, J.D. Buckley, & M.B. Sporn, "Can Dietary Beta-Carotene Materially Reduce Human Cancer Rates?" *Nature*, Vol. 290, March 19, 1981, pp. 201–208.

The Physicians' Health Study (aspirin and beta-carotene), Harvard Medical School, letter to physicians, June 1982.

Pritikin, N., *The Pritikin Program for Diet and Exercise,* New York: Bantam Books, 1981.

Recent Trends in Cancer Deaths, from the National Cancer Institute, *Medical Times,* May 1983, pp. 61–65.

Recommended Dietary Allowances, Vitamin, Mineral, Weight, and Calorie Recommendations, the National Research Council, 9th ed., National Academy of Sciences, 1980.

Seeking Clues to Disease in the Details of Daily Life, the American Cancer Society's Cancer Prevention Study II, Severo, R., *The New York Times,* August 29, 1982, p. 20E.

Shodell, M., "The Intimate Enemy." *Science 82,* September 1982, pp. 46–51.

Sloan, L., and C. Gates, *The 100 Calorie Book,* Los Angeles: Price/Stern/Sloan Publishers, Inc., 1981.

Statistical Bulletin, Metropolitan Life Insurance Company, 1976–80.

Tarnower, H., M.D., and S.S. Baker, *The Complete Scarsdale Medical Diet,* New York: Bantam Books, 1980.

Thomas, L., M.D., *The Youngest Science. Notes of a Medicine-Watcher,* New York: The Viking Press, 1983, pp. 205–206.

"Vitamins and Herbs Are No Bulwark Against an Inadequate Diet": Comments by H.J. Loeffler, Ph.D., to the annual meeting of the California Medical Association, cited in *Internal Medicine News,* June 15–30, 1982, p. 48.

Walker, W.J., M.D., "Changing U.S. Life Style and Declining Vascular Mortality—A Retrospective." (editorial), *New England Journal of Medicine,* Vol. 308, No. 11, March 17, 1983, pp. 649–51.

Weiss, E.S., and R.P. Wolfson, *Cholesterol Counter,* New York: Pyramid Books, 1973.

Woodruff, D.S., Ph.D., *Can You Live to Be 100?,* New York: Signet Books, 1979.

Young, J.H., Ph.D., "Laetrile in Historical Perspective." *Connecticut Medicine,* Vol. 43, No. 8, August 1979, pp. 497–500.

The following sources have also been very helpful:
• *Vital Statistics of the United States.*

143

- U.S. National Center for Health Statistics and U.S. Bureau of the Census.
- National Cancer Institute.
- *World Health Statistics Annual.*
- Department of Health, Education, and Welfare (NIH), cited in *Ca-A Cancer Journal for Clinicians: Cancer Statistics*, January/February issue, annually.
- *Journal of the National Cancer Institute:* "Cancer Incidence and Mortality Trends in the United States: 1935–1974"; "Trends in Cancer Incidence and Mortality in the United States, 1969–1976."
- American Cancer Society, *1980 Cancer Facts and Figures.*
- U.S. Department of Health, Education, and Welfare (Public Health Service), *Health: United States 1979.*
- American Cancer Society, *Cancer Statistics, 1980*, cited in *Cancer in the United States: Is There an Epidemic?* A report by the American Council on Science and Health.

INDEX

Beta-carotene, effects on diet (*cont.*)
  promotion, 132–33, 135
  red palm oil, 134–35
  research fields, 132
  research questions, 136
  resilience of body, 138
  retinol binding protein, 135
  serum studies, 133
  toxicity of vitamin A, 135
Beta units, 61–62, 81–82
BHT, 128
Body chemistry, changing of, and
    cancer risk
  beta-carotene, 127
  estrogens, 127
  overnutrition, 127
  selenium, 127
  vitamin A, 127
  vitamin E, 127
  women, 127–28

C

Cafeteria scoop, for measuring
    vegetables, 81
Calories, defined, 14. *See also*
    Carbohydrates; Diet; Fats;
    Weight loss.
Cancer. *See also* Statistics;
    Symptoms.
  cases of
    breast, 38–39
    delays in treating, dangers of,
      39–41
    lung, 39
    rectal, 39
  history of
    ancient, 42
    chimney sweeps, 42
    factors, 43
    geography, 43
    radium paint, 42–43
  by organs, 118–20
    list, 118–19
    percentage elimination by diet,
      119–20
  regional differences, 28

Cancer. *See also* Statistics;
  Symptoms (*cont.*)
  steps of
    classifications, 37
    and DNA, 35, 36
    initiation, 35
    latency, 35
    oncogenes, 37
    patterns, 37
    promotion, 35–36
    self-repair of DNA, 37
    spread, 37
    transposons, 37
Carbohydrates, 13, 20, 66, 109
  diet, 66, 109
  nature, 13
  needs for, 20
Carcinogens, inhibitors of, 116
Carcinoma, 37
Centicals, 78
Cholesterol, 14, 67, 76, 104, 136
  diet, 67
  foods rich in, 76
  fraction, 136
  science background, 104
Coffee, 115

D

Daily menu, master plan
  breakfast, 94
  dinner, 95
  lunch, 95
  snacks, 94, 95
Diet books
  Atkins diet, 8–9
  Beverly Hills diet, 10–11
  enzymes, 11
  and ketosis, 9
  Pritikin diet, 9
  Scarsdale diet, 9
  special, 8
  and temporary weight loss, 8
  time-oriented, 7–8
Diet, for cancer prevention and
    weight management
  body weight, 65, 66
  calories, 65–66, 67

146